Menopause Mind Shifts

Menopause Mind Shifts

How to break free from your past

and embrace your future.

Debbie van Dijk

Published and distributed in the UK by Amazon Kindle Publishing

Copyright 2023 by Debbie van Dijk

The moral rights of the author have been asserted.

All rights reserved. No part of this book may be reproduced by any mechanical, photographic, or electronic process or in the form of a phonographic recording; nor may it be stored in a retrieval system, transmitted or otherwise be copied for public or private use, other than for 'fair use' as a brief quotation embodied in articles, reviews, without permission of the author.

The information in this book should not be treated as a substitute for professional medical advice; always consult your medical practitioner. Any use of information in this book is at the reader's discretion and risk. Neither the author nor the publisher can be held responsible for any loss, claim, or damage arising from the use or misuse of the suggestions made, the failure to take medical advice, or any material on third-party websites.

ISBN 9798861423311

"Life is not measured by the number of breaths we take, but by the number of moments that take our breath away."

(Anonymous)

The Dragonfly

Front cover photo: By Becky Kelly

Meaning: Hope, change, love

Dragonflies can be a symbol of self that comes with maturity. They can symbolise going past self-created illusions that limit our growth and ability to change.

In many cultures, the dragonfly is seen as a symbol of good luck, prosperity, happiness and new beginnings.

Seize the day, be grateful for what you have, and take that all important leap of faith when you feel the calling to do so.

For my Mum and Dad

I understand so much more

&

I love you both so much.

Contents

Introduction	1
How to approach this book	17
Why write this book?	21
PART ONE IMPLEMENT THESE THINGS NOW	35
Where do you live?	37
Oh, for a good night's Sleep.	39
Move that body!	42
The Hormone Links	45
PART TWO YOUR HISTORY OF DEVELOPMENT	55
Step 1: Understanding who you are	58
Step 2: Let's discover your values.	62
Step 3: Discover your beliefs.	66

Step 4: Speak Your Truth	74
Step 5: How does this affect your menopause journey?	79
PART THREE CONNECTION	81
PART FOUR YOUR COACHING JOURNEY	95
Step 6: Discovering Your Ideal Self	98
Step 7: Overcoming Fear	102
Step 8: Becoming Selfish	111
Step 9: Developing Generosity	122
Step 10: Embracing Uncertainty	134
Step 11: Seeing the bigger picture	137
PART FIVE LETTER TO THE KIDS	143
PART SIX ASCENSION MEDITATION	159
PART SEVEN A WOMEN'S ADVICE	191
Conclusion	195
Resources	203
Acknowledgements	205
About The Author	211

About Soul Decisions Coaching 215

Other Titles by Soul Decisions Coaching 218

Introduction

Menopause is coming out of the closet, and so it should! Although it still feels like we have a long way to go to normalise the conversations and increase awareness and knowledge for many women. It seems my generation is willing and able to contribute and communicate what is needed. For our daughters, sons, husbands, and each other. My research on the subject has taken me far and wide around the globe and has certainly been an enlightening experience. The way in which women were treated in the past was, in most parts, barbaric! It was troubling to read, and it made me angry and terribly sad. I am now a member of different groups

INTRODUCTION

and have many books on the subject, so I feel more connected and open to the topic than when I first started to experience my own menopause journey and did not realise it. Eight years ago, it was definitely not a topic discussed openly or even acknowledged. Not by my GP or the Gynaecology consultant I saw for the issues I was having at the time.

I could not and did not know how to ask for help. A key factor for many women.

Menopause is the right of passage for the next stage in our lives. I could not understand why life had to be so tough when, like childbirth, our bodies are designed to experience it and know what to do. I truly believed in my body when I had my first child. I believed so strongly that my body knew exactly what to do to grow a gorgeous little baby and deliver her into this world safe and healthy. My body knew what to do as I went through puberty, and so did yours.

MENOPAUSE MIND SHIFTS

On reflection, I now see how my childhood had a negative impact on my teenage years and my menopause years. Fear, scarcity, poverty, desperation, abandonment, shame, dependency, embarrassment, worthlessness, lack of trust, anxiety, and not feeling loved all played a significant part in my childhood. I had unknowingly brought those into menopause with me. How was that possible when I had done so much self-development work? How was that possible when my life was great? I have a fabulous husband, amazing kids, loads of love in our home, and so much more. It was a real dichotomy. My life was great, yet inside, I felt pain, suffering and loss.

Our bodies are miraculous. We are miraculous. Why was this thing called menopause completely knocking me off my feet emotionally, physically, and psychologically? Why do we take our bodies for granted and abuse them in so many ways, often unknowingly?

INTRODUCTION

It got me thinking about lifestyles pre-menopause and the realisation that however you have lived your life then impacts your journey through menopause. If from your childhood you have some strong limiting beliefs, if you are not living or knowing your values, if you are surrounding yourself with people who drag you down, if you are people pleasing or stuck in a victim role, if old habits no longer serve you, then your menopause journey will have added difficulties for you to navigate. If your childhood had a fair amount of trauma in it, then you will bring that too.

Now, as a Life Coach, my current interest lies in the way our minds and bodies connect during this turbulent (for some) season of our lives. How do our past experiences affect our menopause journey? How do our minds, our thoughts, contribute to the experience we have? Could this emotional roller coaster be prevented with a better approach and more tools at hand?

Yes, it can.

MENOPAUSE MIND SHIFTS

After working with many women over the past ten years and having experienced my own turbulent menopause journey, I realised for some of us that our past appears in our present to rock our lives back and forth, often tipping us over. That is, until we do something to heal ourselves within.

We are all shaped by the significant emotional events that occur in our lives from childhood to adulthood. Some of which we remember, some we don't. What I have come to realise, especially over the past few years working with many women and as my own menopause journey unfolded, is the importance of what we have carried through life with us up to this point. Our thinking habits, the roles we play, what we value, what we believe, what we fear, what we regret, what we choose, and how we act and react. Who we are being or comparing ourselves to. Who we spend time with. How we live day to day. How we have loved. What we fear. What we procrastinate on. What we sabotage. Our self-talk.

INTRODUCTION

All of this comes through menopause with us if we allow it.

I acknowledge that women, in general, feel that they must be seen to be coping. With everything!!! They can't possibly go easy on themselves, or they would lose face in front of others. Others could be anyone, but especially other women. The comparisons we fall into in our younger years can, and often do, plague our adulthood.

Are we, as women, our own worst critics?

Alas, I think we might be! We certainly can be.

It appears we are quite good at self-criticism and being critical of each other. This is something I have found interesting as I have grown. I believe that women need women. Who else can fully understand the wiring of a woman's body and emotions than another woman? It was such a relief when, through my own journey of releasing my childhood subconscious feelings of neglect, abandonment, scarcity, and fear-based thinking, my menopause symptoms eased dramatically. I had a great poverty story running riot in my head, often paralysing me that wasn't even my story. I was stuck in not feeling enough. I was the fixer of all things. Drama found its way to me so I could solve it for others. I was a true hero for the wrong reasons. The thing was, it was all hidden within. I didn't understand it. I felt lost and alone and couldn't understand what to do or where to go. When I gained the awareness and sought help, I was able to drop that self-righteous, judgmental (although based in fear) side of myself that once existed. (Yes, I must admit I used to have quite a lot of very strong opinions about things that had absolutely nothing to do with me!!)

The lack of understanding of the changes our bodies go through and how this can be linked to and affected by our childhood traumas was so fascinating to me. I was experiencing it all first-hand, and somehow, inside, I knew it was linked, and I could do something about it. I observed women (my

INTRODUCTION

clients, friends, and family members in my ancestral line) pushing themselves to diet, to go hard out on exercise as if they were in their twenties again. To continuously put others' needs first, ignoring their own. It was as if I could see the loss, pain and grief in their eyes and hearts because I understood it firsthand. Exhausting themselves. What for? What was the point?

A life truly well-lived is not about the amount of money we have, the status we carry, the car we drive or any material possessions. In truth, these things can be very lonely, as well as being great to have. A truly well-lived life is abundant in love, kindness, connection, knowing you are enough just for being you, and so much more that money and material possessions just cannot match.

When our life experiences that cause us pain are felt, expressed and let go of, then we are better equipped to understand, to love and cherish ourselves, to treat ourselves better and to show others how we want to be treated as we go through menopause with all its trials and tribulations. We lessen the burden we carry at a time in our lives when we possibly need it most—an easier road to travel if you can shed the pain of your past. The only way to do this is to acknowledge, feel through it and let go with forgiveness.

When better understood, we have the option to make informed choices that are often different to the habitual choices we would have made. It becomes a positive turning point in our lives at a time when life is changing for us anyway as we age. For me, it was a transformational journey that, at one time, I could never have conceived. Understanding and learning a new way of being then helps us gain some level of clarity. A point at which we can take some power back into our own hands, hearts, minds, and bodies. I found it all very liberating. The coaching through menopause journey filled me with courage and confidence that I wasn't stuck and would feel well again one day. I certainly wasn't going to die as I

INTRODUCTION

sometimes felt, and even at my weakest and most vulnerable, I was never giving up on the life I wanted for myself. A life that was rich with love, positivity, fun, happiness, connections, courage, and so much more.

I chose life. I decided I was worth it. Most importantly, I decided my life was worth paying attention to.

As a life coach who has worked with many women, I became so aware of the detrimental impact not knowing and living our values and living with limiting subconscious beliefs has on our menopause years. What I experienced with clients was the way negative attitudes and limiting beliefs affected their ability to cope with menopause symptoms. Childhood experiences and early adult experiences altered and limited my client's abilities to let go, see things from a different perspective, look after themselves first, and allow calmness to enter their lives. Defining moments from childhood formed who they were in the world. Created beliefs formed to protect themselves as children, shaped their adult behaviour. Allowing self-care was not an option. Shrinking themselves, hiding their true self in the shadows, and not allowing others to see or help was the choice of the day, the week, the month, the year. A perpetual cycle set in well before menopause came along and then exacerbated by menopause symptoms.

This book intends to highlight the importance of mind shifts and emotional trauma identification and release as we navigate the turbulent waters of menopause and to give you the direction in which to steer your menopausal mind shift ship. I wanted to sail my ship on peaceful still waters with bright blue skies and the sun beaming down on me as I bathed in its luxurious warmth and vibrancy as I aged! I got there eventually, but it took some time to figure it out and to remain true to myself. True to what I wanted out of my life. I still remind myself of what I want. It's a continuous journey through life.

INTRODUCTION

To master this, I had to pay attention to feeling and expressing my emotions. It was a journey of searching, discovering, and cherishing those things that made a positive difference and pushing, pulling, wailing, drowning in the unknown waters and turbulent winds of a mass of symptoms I didn't know were menopause and the link to emotions I didn't know were present. Putting down the anchor (being still) and staying true to what was working in the moment, releasing the sails, and letting go. Trusting my mind and body became a real challenge that, instinctively, I just knew I could challenge right back if I could muster up the energy somehow. Being defeated by menopause as my mother was, I would not consider it an option. Allowing the next breeze of information to take me where I needed to go was my choice, even when I did not know the destination.

I began to trust myself. I committed to trusting my evolving cargo of tools and offloading those that no longer served me. This did mean letting go of some relationships, a job I absolutely loved, having tough conversations, hiding away, and taking a stern look at myself, my actions, and my reactions. Ultimately, I had to make different choices, and at the time, that was strongly connected to my fear of not surviving menopause. Of growing old too quickly. Of never feeling youthful, sexy, vibrant. Of never feeling enough!

Like many, many women I know and have read stories from, there was simply a time when I felt like I was dying. I know that sounds dramatic to some, and believe me, I am not a dramatic person. I prefer not to have drama in my life, but I just had nothing left in the tank. Nothing left to give. Depleted! I was desperate to find the high-energy, fun, go-getting, absolutely loving life gal I knew I was inside. I knew she must be in there somewhere. It was shocking, to say the least when she was nowhere to be found. I was swimming in the darkness of anxiety and paralysing fear. My energy and zest for life had disappeared.

INTRODUCTION

I once heard Tony Robins say, "Getting through anything in life is 20% mechanics and 80% psychology". The 80% is where you make the shift. Having experienced working with women and my own mindset, I can say I truly believe this statement to be true. Even in my darkest moments, if I could get my head around something or, better still, 'let go' of what was going on in my head. If I could look at all perspectives and stay open to possibilities or simply allow myself to let go, whether I liked it or not, I was 80% of the way there.

So how do you do that when, quite honestly, your menopause experience is totally devastating your life, and you feel like you are dying emotionally, spiritually, psychologically, and physically!!!!!

Please believe me in this moment that you can. By discovering, accepting, loving and being yourself. By being the best you you can possibly be on a daily basis. Moment by moment. When you learn this, your life will change for the better. You cannot do this alone. I cannot stress that enough. We are born for connection and connect we must do if we are to be truly healthy. I have always believed 'women need women' and we need each other even more as we go through significant life stages.

How did I do it?

I did the work of discovering myself, attending the courses, feeling the pain, and acknowledging what was holding me hostage. I committed to be fully responsible for my own life.

Now, above everything else, I prioritise my peace. (Thank you, Ascension Meditation.)

I will show you how you can do this as we go through the book.

From my heart and soul to yours, with so much love to you on your journey

Happy reading, Deb xx

How to approach this book

'Here is the theme: 'Supremely Gentle.'

We live in a world of busyness. Full speed ahead seems to be how most people approach life. I remember a time when in my head I would often scream the word STOP followed by 'I want to get off' followed by 'I need to get out of here' followed by and spoken a little more quietly, 'help'.

So, when I sat to write this book, I thought it would be good to give it a theme.

HOW TO APPROACH THIS BOOK

Thank you, Mahakala Ishaya, for the gift of these very special words. 'Supremely gentle'. I heard these words many times during Ascension meditation training. As I sat peacefully, waiting for the theme of the book to reveal itself, this beautiful reminder came to me. 'Be supremely gentle.'

As you are sat now reading, take a nice, slow, deep breath. Maybe another? Another?

Now read on, beautiful soul; we have things to discover.

Your approach

Approaching this book with wonder and curiosity will be more beneficial to your outcome than going through it beating yourself up because you think you should already know some of this stuff, you've already been through some of this learning, or it highlights areas in your life that create painful emotion.

MENOPAUSE MIND SHIFTS

Be curious as to why, as an adult, you might be stuck in certain ways of thinking or stuck in certain emotions as they bubble to the surface for you. Curiosity is a wonderful way to approach life.

Be curious and wonder how you could possibly think differently about the situation now as the adult that you are.

If you can find a life coach to help you explore, even better. We all need help at some point in our lives, and the perspective of others is truly a gift to yourself. This is not a journey to take alone. Believe me. I tried, and it does not work. It is also not a journey that needs to be filled with sadness and reliving trauma. It is a journey that can be exciting, uplifting, and fulfilling. Why? Because it is a journey of your beautiful, precious life.

Most of all, be gentle in your approach and slow life down enough to give yourself the space just to be. Can I repeat that for you? Be gentle in your approach and slow down enough to give yourself the space just to be.

Your future self will be so grateful.

Resources at the back of the book

There are some wonderful books out there that will give you detailed information about physical symptoms and how to cope, HRT, and women's stories. I have a list of them at the back of the book for you. I've enjoyed all of them; they have been a great resource while researching this book.

I want to give you permission right now to prioritise your own peace, your own health, and your own life.

Why write this book?

The purpose of writing this book is for women like my mum, whose mental and emotional health deteriorated beyond recognition through her menopause years.

My mum is a beautiful, kind, loving and courageous woman who had a terrible, poverty-stricken, abusive childhood. She must have lived in paralysing fear throughout her childhood and early adulthood. She was one of 13; her dad was abusive, and her mum died young. She married my dad when pregnant with my older sister. Forced to marry (I'm not sure?), they had to live in her childhood home with all her brothers and sisters.

WHY WRITE THIS BOOK?

They soon had me and then, two years later, my younger sister.

Money was scarce, but somehow, they managed to move into a new house. I imagine that it felt like a palace to her. A dream come true. For a very short period of time, she had three happy little girls, a husband, a lovely home with a vegetable garden and her own kitchen to bake in. Being the homemaker was something she loved, as well as growing food in our garden to bring into the kitchen to cook. Teaching us, showing us what it was like to have a stable, loving home even though this was short-lived.

One day, disaster struck; the house was taken from them, and our safe life was gone.

Dad too. No explanation. Just gone out of our lives. He never returned to live with us.

Our bags packed, belongings on the street, we carried our things back to Mum's childhood home.

MENOPAUSE MIND SHIFTS

Back into the poverty, the abuse she had known for most of her life. The three of us marching along the street, heading into the unknown, feeling the heaviness of the trauma that was unfolding.

Our lives were shattered by the experience. Fear and devastation well and truly set into our little bodies.

Mum has never recovered from the deep-rooted traumatic experiences in her life. When she started to go through menopause, I distinctly remember her taking a turn for the worse. One day, she collapsed in the kitchen. After that, I have images of her sitting in front of the fire, drinking from bottles of perfume and alcohol. Rocking back and forth, cigarette in hand, gazing at the fire lost somewhere inside herself. Nobody coming to help.

Her menopause journey was all the worse for the experiences she had prior to it. Exacerbated by menopause symptoms and no strategies, coping mechanisms or being in the right environment to cope or seek help. Her three girls far too young to even begin to understand or know what to do.

My sister recently said that she hated that she has been unable to help Mum more. What I know is that when you come from a place of hurt, pain and devastation yourself, there is only so much you can do with the resources and knowledge you have. This is true for any of us in any situation. Any of you beautiful women reading this who feel hurt, sadness, abandonment, grief, loss, regret, shame, you can only do and be what you alone are capable of in any given moment. I know and understand this place. It is dark, and you feel like you are never going to come out of it. If this is you, I'm sending you all my love right here in this sentence. I want to tell you that it is possible. Be kind, compassionate and loving towards yourself. It is in the being that we can heal. No blame towards yourself or others will ease any of the pain you might feel about certain circumstances in your life. Blame is pointless.

Pain, regret, guilt, shame, and fear will never create good health, yet these are the emotions I see people living time and time again. So, if you carry these and focus on them whilst also going through the hormonal upheaval of menopause, can you see how much more debilitating your health will be? I absolutely believe that had Mum had the kind of help that I write about in this book, then her life would have been profoundly better.

> *"You can only do what you know in any given moment of your life with the resources you have available at the time."*

A day from my childhood

"It's another Sunday morning, I'm eight years old. It's quite early, and I know he is not going to be here for hours, but I choose to sit at the window looking and waiting for him to arrive. Today, he might turn up! Today, he might turn up early! So, I sit and wait. Morning turns to lunchtime, and he

WHY WRITE THIS BOOK?

still hasn't arrived. If I go to see if there is any food in the house, I will miss his arrival, and then he might think I don't care. That he is not the most important thing in my entire life. That I live for these Sundays when he might or might not arrive to take us away from this hell hole, even if only for a few hours.

So, I sit, and I wait. Alone.

I don't remember if my sisters sat with me.

Lunchtime turns to evening, and I will not leave my seat until it goes dark, for then I know for certain he will not be coming.

He does not arrive.

He must have something on. Something more important.'"

This is one of the experiences from my childhood that continuously fed the feelings of abandonment, rejection, not being worthy or enough, and not feeling loved. Week after week.

Client's story

I want to share a client story with you that illustrates how our childhoods shape our lifestyles.

One conversation went like this:

"Are you going through menopause?"

Client – "Yes."

"How do you know?"

Client – "I feel like shit, and I had some bloods done."

"What are your main symptoms?"

Client – "Pain in all my joints and totally exhausted all the time. Seem to feel anxious often and can't multi-task anymore because I lose my train of thought. My brain feels foggy, and I have put so much weight on."

"What do you do to look after yourself?"

Client – "I go to the gym at 5am 5 times a week for a 1-hour workout before I go to work.

Breakfast?

Client – "Coffee, I don't have time to eat."

"How many hours do you work?"

Client – "Between 40-50, depending on what is needed. Sometimes 60, and that can be all hours of the day or night."

Do you work weekends?

Client – "Yes, I work most weekends, or I'm on call."

"Why do you work so many hours?"

Client – "I need to support others as they have been going through a tough time."

"How long has this been going on for?"

Client – "Oh, years. I just now feel like I have nothing left to give. I used to be able to cope, but my body doesn't want to anymore.

"What do you want?"

Client – "I don't know anymore!"

This beautiful woman came to me when she was desperate, about to have a nervous breakdown, had lost any passion for a profession she had loved and was exceptionally good at, was losing her hair, damaging her relationships, she had black puffy circles under her eyes and looked exhausted. Her whole body was in such pain that she had to take regular pain medication, which had stopped having effect. She has no time for herself, her husband, or the kids. No joy. No fun. No relaxation. Just overwhelming exhaustion.

WHY WRITE THIS BOOK?

Where did that fierce work ethic, being responsible for others, being the hero, saving everyone else, pushing her body to extreme limits, and neglecting her own needs and health come from?

As we delved deeper, I discovered her dad left them when she was very small, and her mum worked three jobs to keep the roof over their head. Her aunties were a significant part of her childhood, all very strong women. From a very early age, she had been taught to be strong, independent, work hard, and push herself. She admired all the women in her life and quite right what amazing role models. Yet somewhere along the line, she had misinterpreted some of the lessons. She could still be strong, independent, be committed to her work. What her body was telling her to do was stop the pushing. The pushing is making you ill. The pushing is taking your health and vitality and even more so now that you are going through menopause.

Be strong, of course; just be it with a soft and gentle approach.

Now, when you take the PUSH (which she was, which comes from a lack of self-worth, old beliefs and not-enoughness) and more into menopause with you, watch out!! You are in for a tough ride, and your family will join you.

I was elated when, after only a few short months of working with this lady, her whole life turned around. She found her peace and stillness; her approach to life became supremely gentle, gently committed to her work, gym workouts not as aggressive, and spending more time with her husband and kids without guilt that she was relaxing.

What did she do? She went through my Life Coaching and Bowen Therapy program with me, and she learnt Ascension meditation. A powerful, beautiful, life-changing combination. She's not the only one.

WHY WRITE THIS BOOK?

I am as guilty of the above things as the next woman, so I was elated when I discovered how to overcome them.

Is my life 100% better for my discoveries? Heck yes, absolutely, without a shadow of a doubt, and so are my clients!

It's all a journey. A magical journey of your precious, precious life, ladies. I love that you have bought this book. I love that you want to find your own answers, and I love that you can pass your knowledge down to your own daughters, nieces, daughters-in-law, and even your sons, and let's not forget husbands (more for them later). You and only you can decide it is time for change.

Change is possible when you believe it.

Where do I start?

So, where do you start if you want to change? You start with a solid, unrelenting commitment to your own health, and you do not let anyone interfere. You prioritise your own peace in this lifetime. Everyone deserves that. You deserve that, and you do for yourself first what you would normally do for others. You are the priority. If you do this for yourself, you are helping everyone else anyway. You will shine your own light in order to show others how to shine theirs.

The right time to do this?

NOW

xx

PART ONE

IMPLEMENT THESE

THINGS NOW

You can read and read and gather tons of information to the point of being overwhelmed, but if you don't implement any of it, it becomes just information gathering. I know that you could flick through the book and choose different chapters, so I decided to put my first three impactful actions at the front of the book. Here for you to choose to start right away. Change is your choice, and as my beautiful friend Aditi says....

PART ONE
IMPLEMENT THESE THINGS NOW

"When we believe change is possible, change happens."

Aditi Ishaya

Where do you live?

Where do you live? Above the line or below the line? When I was first introduced to this, it did wonders for keeping me (and the kids) on track. To be honest, it was a bit of a blow to me when I realised I was spending most of my time below the line. I had to remind myself that I had given myself permission to be 'supremely gentle' in my approach as I recognised my relationship with each word from below the line. As you do this for yourself, give yourself the gift and permission to do the same. It is only with awareness that we can choose an alternative way of being.

Do you live here, **Above the Line?**

Accountability, Responsibility, Ownership.

Be solution-focused. Take action. Believe in self. Live with intention.

Or do you live here, **Below the Line?**

Blame. Excuses. Justification. Denial. Anger.

PART ONE
IMPLEMENT THESE THINGS NOW

Wait for others, compare yourself to others, take on the victim role.

This is not an exhaustive list, but I think you see the picture that develops when you choose where you live! We will thread these themes throughout the book, so more on this later. For now, be curious about where you live and why. Whenever possible and always being gentle with yourself, keep yourself above the line. Life is so much more abundant, positive, and fun when you do. There is also a strength and confidence that begins to develop and grow within as you stay above the line and take full responsibility for your life. Awareness of this is a great start.

Oh, for a good night's Sleep.

During menopause, our sleep patterns can go crazy as our hormones spike and plummet. This could be due to hot flushes, aching joints, a racing mind, anxiety, body pain, or someone snoring next to you. I'm sure if you have been reading all about menopause, you will know how vital a good night's sleep is to help you cope with the symptoms experienced. This section is to get you to implement NOW. Here are some top tips. Small steps make such a difference.

1) Start going to bed half an hour earlier than you usually would. This means eating earlier (very important) to keep insulin lower before you go to bed. When you have done that for a week, increase it to an hour.

2) Have your room cool/cold and a weighted blanket on top of you. (This goes back to our primal days and links with our rhythm for sleep, which is

PART ONE
IMPLEMENT THESE THINGS NOW

that our core temperature drops and our nervous system calms when our bodies are weighted down.)

3) When you get into bed. Sit up in a comfortable position and breathe slowly. If you know some breathing techniques, use them; if not, breathe slowly and gently. When you feel ready, lie down and continue slow and gentle breathing.

"A beautiful day begins with a beautiful mindset. When you wake up, take a second to think about what a privilege it is to simply be alive and healthy. The moment you start acting like life is a blessing, I assure you it will start to feel like one. Time spent appreciating is a time worth living."

Unknown

4) Setting your circadian rhythm starts in the morning, so when you wake up, allow the day's light into your eyes for 10 to 20 minutes. You might go for a walk or stand at the window or door with your

morning cuppa. Breathe in the fresh air, look around you, and enjoy the calmness of the morning.

PART ONE
IMPLEMENT THESE THINGS NOW

Move that body!

Aching joints and stiffness can be a real problem during menopause. Morning and evening stretch and strengthening exercises are essential to your daily routine. Even a 5-minute routine will make a difference in how you feel. Our bodies are designed to move. So, let's get moving.

You can Google many simple routines or gain advice from an expert in this area, paying specific attention to your menopausal body and what it needs. Walking is fabulous. You are not only getting exercise but also out in nature. The aim is always gentleness. Why? Because your body is under so much stress and inflammation anyway, you do not want to add to this.

A great morning routine could be getting up earlier, doing some stretches, meditation time, or quiet time to allow your body to adjust to the day ahead.

MENOPAUSE MIND SHIFTS

"Remember, when we believe change is possible, change happens."

The Hormone Links

Menopause hormone shifts play havoc with our daily lives. I realise how much I took my body for granted and how it never occurred to me the importance of each of the hormones that kept my body in good health and vitality until they were depleted or, worse, gone. In her book 'Menopause Reset' Dr. Mindy Pelz writes about our hormones having a hierarchy. Here is a summary of what she tells us:

'Oxytocin is the top of the hierarchy, the best hormone that boosts our feelings of love and connection, and when you get lots of it, you experience a major benefit in your health.'

THE HORMONE LINKS

Cortisol is next. This hormone can have a huge detrimental effect on your health and, unfortunately, rules daily life for many in the rushing, pushing, packed schedules of life as we know it today. It is the hormone responsible for giving and maintaining belly fat, spikes your blood sugar, and wakes you frequently during the night as a stress response. Oh, joy!

Insulin comes up next. This hormone is released from the pancreas when we eat. If we eat lots of sugar, we will produce more insulin. If we eat lots of carbohydrates, we will produce more insulin. Whatever your body cannot use, it will store as fat. As we know, the fat stored and gained can be very difficult to shift during menopause.

Can you see that by knowing a little about these hormones, you can create some positive solutions in your behaviour from your past to your present? For example, boost your Oxytocin by having more fun with loved ones and friends—more time with your animals and out in nature. Or help to calm your cortisol levels by learning a meditation technique, sitting quietly, breathing slowly, moving your body gently, being kinder to yourself, and stopping the rushing in your life. Reduce insulin levels by learning to fast between meals, lowering the carbs and sugars in your diet, and eating at more appropriate times.

I realise now how dominant cortisol has been for most of my life. How the traumatic childhood experiences kept me in fight or flight, feeling unsafe even when this was not the truth in my adult life. My inner world did not know it, and I suspect many people experience the same. There was a time when I forgot how to have fun because I was so wrapped up in work and responsibility that I could not find time or energy to do anything nice for myself.

What did this do?

It kept cortisol high and oxytocin low. I did not know this at the time. Life was one big push, and I remember referring to life as being 'hard.' Asking myself, 'Why is life always so hard?'

The following hormones to mention are what I consider to be the most obviously thought of when we begin our menopause journey: estrogen, progesterone, and testosterone, our sex hormones. What a merry dance (well, no, not really!!) these hormones take us on. Dr. Pelz tells us that progesterone going low during menopause is a result of the stress we experience in our 30s and 40s. What!!

Dropping progesterone causes us to feel uneasy and anxious at the slightest thing or nothing at all. Have you experienced that? I remember sitting in a cafe with my friend and having a lovely time. Unexpectedly, I began to feel a dreaded sense of fear creeping its way up my body as if a full-blown panic attack was about to grip me. The amount of fear and anxiety I felt in that moment shook me to my core—unexplainable fear.

MENOPAUSE MIND SHIFTS

Estrogen and progesterone work together, and if one is out of balance, they are both out of balance. Testosterone gives us our sex drive, motivates us, and helps us build muscle. When that drops during menopause, we are left with low libido, flabby muscles, and reduced motivation. Not pleasant experiences, for sure.

We can deduce from this information that our daily habits and lives need an overhaul.

Change is afoot!

Will you approach this chapter as a possibility for change and give your life and health the attention it needs to age well and live well?

The hormone shift we experience through menopause can be brutal, planting us firmly on an emotional roller coaster ride that we would rather not take. For many women, this creates a time for re-evaluating life completely. Leaving marriages in search of something calmer, more peaceful, something for oneself, maybe? Feeling less tolerant? Wanting to get away from all the noise and expectations of others?

Wanting to get out of here, leave, run away. Does this sound familiar? 'I just need to get out '. I remember saying this to my husband in a moment of desperation. Of not knowing what was happening to me to make me feel such a drastic feeling. I knew logically it wasn't what I wanted to do. I certainly didn't want to leave him or the life we had built with our amazing kids. I didn't want to leave my soul mate, but I did want to leave. It felt so much better to share the fear of such a strong statement.

Are we going crazy? Are we losing our minds? For some women, the answer is yes. Though through my own experience, I am convinced this is not just menopause, but our traumatic life experiences that contribute to our ability to cope with the changes that menopause brings. This is one reason why I know we can do so much more for ourselves during this time.

Releasing the trauma, mending relationships, and focusing more on our mental and emotional health as well as our physical health. Redefining how we want to be treated by others and how we treat ourselves. It is all possible when you know how. When you figure out what is right for you and when you clear the trauma you hold in your own body. When you can allow those irrational thoughts to be there. To stop and, with gentleness, allow them to be there, knowing that you will pull through them. They are not permanent.

Trauma trapped in the body can reveal itself in many ways. It can be pain felt in your heart, the thoughts that loop over and over through your mind, the knots in your stomach, repeated illnesses, the tightening in your throat when you want to speak and can't get the words out, the irrational responses to what can be insignificant comments, the trying to prove you are right and someone else is wrong, having to know everything about everything even though this is impossible. The list goes on and on.

Trauma trapped in your body prevents you from living your own life. Choosing joy and peace over fear is difficult because we may not think we are worthy. Being trapped in fear disables you from embracing joy and happiness, keeping you in a cage of sadness and grief. This is not always obvious sometimes; it can be subtle.

In the hundreds of clients and patients I have worked with over the past 30 years, both through my business and the health services in New Zealand and the UK, and of the different cultures, acknowledging and experiencing full-blown emotion was not a safe place to be. Acknowledging, experiencing, and expressing emotion was not even considered an option.

Yet, in the release of that emotion lies the solution.

To allow emotion to be present in all its glory and to love yourself and others regardless. To accept that emotion, whatever it is, to rise through you and then leave. Yet the distraction of daily life is welcomed and dominated as if somehow that is easier. Is it?

At the core of our being is love and the shadows of emotional pain.

Can you make peace with that which creates both within you?

If you were to look back on your life at the memories that created your different emotional responses, what would they be?

Let's look at all emotions, not just the sad ones, because all of them make you who you are and the choices you make today. This isn't about doom and gloom. It isn't about staying stuck in painful memories. It is about loving who you are—loving all of you. Loving how you live your life and the choices you make.

You are an adult now, and the memories are in the past, so if you look at the memories from your adult self with a view to loving the younger version of you that experienced those memories, you can give yourself now what you needed at the time.

What did you need at the time?

What is your understanding now?

Think of a memory that keeps coming up for you that is like a loop going around in your mind and heart. It just keeps coming back. There is something very beautiful that happens when you can see this memory from a distance and then, as your adult self, go and support yourself in the memory. Inner child work is very powerful. As the adult that you are now, can you see it from different perspectives?

PART TWO
YOUR HISTORY OF DEVELOPMENT

If your life is not turning out the way you want it to, or there are certain aspects of your life that you are uncomfortable with, then it's time for some discoveries. I would love you to approach this next chapter with genuine curiosity. The generations before us all have an impact on who we are today. We learn so much from our parents, both consciously and subconsciously. Their programming becomes your programming. When something is out

PART TWO
YOUR HISTORY OF DEVELOPMENT

of alignment, we feel it on a deep level. Not always understanding what it is or why. We are constantly evolving, growing, learning, changing and expanding, yet so many of us are locked into how we have been doing things our whole lives. Locked in survival mode. I think Guy Ferdman from Satori Prime puts it well when he says, 'We meddle (meddle/fix it, is our protector pattern) when out of alignment and end up running into survival patterns'—eventually, the loop returns.

We have stories we carry with us. Expectations of ourselves and others are often unrealistic, confirm limiting beliefs and lead to us feeling let down. If we are stuck in expectation, we lose sight of all that we have to be grateful for.

If we stop seeking to change our external world and focus on our internal world, life will become effortless, and an effortless existence is what we all deserve to live—fully immersed in love, peace, joy, and happiness.

MENOPAUSE MIND SHIFTS

So, let's go and discover some stuff.

PART TWO
YOUR HISTORY OF DEVELOPMENT

Step 1: Understanding who you are

Sometimes, I think it is quite a strange concept to ask yourself, 'Who am I?' Actually, I think most people would ask, 'What's life all about?' or 'What's the point?' or 'What am I doing with my life?' If someone was to ask you, who are you? What would you say? Your name? What you do for a living? Mmm, but is that actually you? Or is it what you do? Not who you are. There is a difference, I think.

When we are young, we worry that we don't fit in, and we begin to compare ourselves to others. Obviously, I am not saying everyone does this, but if you have ever felt stuck in your life or you are feeling stuck now, do you find yourself comparing? I know there was a time when I did.

Then, one day, I decided to stop. It was pointless and time-consuming, and it really didn't make me feel good about myself.

It was like a constant reinforcement that I wasn't good enough because I wasn't like such and such a body or I didn't have the material things that they had. I realised the life I had created for myself was actually wonderful. What mattered most to me was that I was healthy, my family was healthy, and we had a wonderful marriage and amazing kids. I also loved my team at work and the work that I was doing. That I was happy with myself. As a family moving to live in another country, we were having an incredible adventure. We had taken risks to make that happen, and I was proud of us for that. The life I had created was completely opposite to my own upbringing. I was proud of that, too.

So, this is me. I love my life. I take risks, and when things don't go the way, I expect them to, I find another way. I'm solution focused. I accept emotion when it comes and don't hold on to it, as it is just a natural part of my being. I love adventure, being out in nature, being aware of the sun's heat on my face and the breeze as it brushes my cheeks.

PART TWO
YOUR HISTORY OF DEVELOPMENT

I love to laugh and sing and dance when anyone is watching. I love to set off on my bike and not know where I'm going. I love to eat well and sleep well because it's so good for you, especially during menopause. I love to stretch my comfort zone. It's scary and fascinating at the same time. I appreciate that life is worth living now, always in this precious moment of time. Love is my number one top value.

I am love.

I am adventure.

I am loyal.

I am courage.

I am fun.

I am connection.

I am this and so much more.

So, who are you? What would you write about yourself? If you don't want to write a paragraph, try starting your sentence, I am… " and then continue to write sentences until you can't think of anything else.

I am……..

PART TWO
YOUR HISTORY OF DEVELOPMENT

Step 2: Let's discover your values.

This is an exercise I love doing face-to-face with clients so that we can discuss their discoveries. It's such a wonderful discovery and has a positive impact on your life when you realise what you truly value. It helps you to understand how you hold yourself back. Which values you are living, and which values you are not. It helps you to understand the difficulties you might be having in relationships. What things you are tolerating that maybe you don't want to tolerate anymore? It helps you to understand your emotions.

Discovering your values is so insightful, and I feel it is the first thing to do when you are searching for some answers, when you don't feel right, and you don't know where to turn.

Our values are a guide for our emotional compass, which can go way off course at times. The mindset we develop from experiences we encounter throughout life travels with us through menopause, bringing many challenges. Let's take a look at some examples:

You are a perfectionist?

You are the clown?

You are the hero?

You are the victim?

You are the pleaser?

You are the rushing woman? (Definition by Dr. Mindy Peltz in Menopause Rest.)

Can you recognise yourself in any of these roles? If you do, is it time to let go and release yourself of the pressure the role creates?

To start to understand yourself better or even to get to know who you are, do the following exercise to discover your values.

PART TWO
YOUR HISTORY OF DEVELOPMENT

Step 1: Choose 20 values from the list below. Write them down.

Compassion, Trust, Wellness, Respect, Family, Kindness, Empathy, Love, Loyalty, Connection, Gratitude, Teamwork, Authenticity, Forgiveness, Integrity, Wisdom, Security, Persistence, Humour, Spirituality, Strength, Open-mindedness, Creativity, Generosity, Knowledge, Leadership, Confidence, Community, Tenacity, Bravery, Beauty, Inclusion, Resilience, Ethics, Independence, Adventure, Self-Growth, Humility, Love of Learning, Collaboration, Courage, Assertiveness, Resourcefulness, Balance, Commitment, Passion, Curiosity, Vitality, Fun, Change, Fairness,

Step 2: Reduce these from 20 to 10. Write them down.

Step 3: Reduce these 10 to 6. Write them down.

Step 4: Write your top 6 in order of priority.

Step 5: Spend time writing about why you have these values and why each individual one is important to you. Take at least 15 minutes per value.

Step 6: Now, with curiosity, ponder on how you live each value daily. Which values are you not living daily? Which values match your partner, your friends? Which ones are a struggle in relationships?

If there are any missing for you, that's ok, just write your own. It's important to know what is true for you. It is important to know the basis on which you live your life.

Now, live these daily and see how your life begins to transform.

PART TWO
YOUR HISTORY OF DEVELOPMENT

Step 3: Discover your beliefs.

Understanding that we all have different perspectives on life and accepting that others have different opinions and are allowed to be so can also have a freeing effect on our lives. How many times have you tried to convince someone of your way of thinking only to be disappointed that you cannot talk them around? Or that relationships have suffered because you believe something so strongly that it does not connect with what someone else believes? Maybe even full-scale angry outbursts have occurred.

Have you heard the phrase or even said the phrase, 'I will believe it when I see it?' What if you didn't then see it? Would you still believe whatever it is to be a possibility? The Satori Prime brothers helped me to think of this in a different way. What if you believe it and then you will see it? I personally much prefer this way of looking at this phrase. If I believe something, it usually materialises. So, if I believe it, then it's just a case of waiting for it to appear. Lovely. Fun perspective. I like that.

Our belief system is shaped by the experiences we have throughout our lives. It has the potential to change over time as we age, mature, grow, and learn new things from life and relationships. Sometimes, actually often, we have blind spots. Our beliefs can either empower us or keep us stuck. We become stuck in limiting beliefs and limited thinking. Our minds will always find evidence in our surroundings to prove what we believe. All of which are there to 'keep us safe.'

Have you experienced this with your children? Do you believe they should behave a certain way? They have a different idea. You try to convince them; they don't want to listen? They want to go their own way and discover their own path, and we struggle to let go and trust that they will be safe.

This happens, doesn't it? Is it just me? As the nest becomes empty and menopause is well and truly set

PART TWO
YOUR HISTORY OF DEVELOPMENT

in, our kids are now young adults transitioning into adulthood, experiencing their own hormonal upheaval. We are all finding the courage to let go and grow from the emotional experience of what we once believed and transforming into mature adult to adult with healthy, reciprocal relationships. Healthy relationships with ourselves.

I understand this does not always happen. Relationships are complex. We are complex. Reciprocal relationships are limited in our lifetime.

Now is the time to revamp our lives, discover our values, discover our beliefs, rid ourselves of limitations, and fully embrace this wonderful stage of life. Doing this for ourselves first and foremost and doing this for the now young adults we have brought into this world.

I also understand that not all of us have children. What I would say here is never underestimate your impact on those around you. We have wonderful, cherished friendships who don't have children of their own, and what I see is how much of an impact they have on everyone around them. Young and old.

So, to create new beliefs, we first look at our current beliefs to see if they need a revamp.

This takes some inward reflection. Please complete the following sentence with the first words that come to you: (do not overthink it.)

I always...

I am...

They are...

We are...

I can't...

I can...

I must...

My life is...

PART TWO
YOUR HISTORY OF DEVELOPMENT

Can you see any negativity in what you have written? This is your opportunity to re-write any of the above beliefs that do not serve you in a positive way or that do not match what you value.

Take some time to reflect on each belief. How does it make you feel? Where do you feel the sensation in your body?

Stomach – Fear

Chest – Sadness

Neck – Anxiety/Fear

Shoulders – Frustration

Allow the sensation to be expressed and released. Your body wants to release any imbalances you feel from your discoveries, so allow this to happen. Remember to be supremely gentle with yourself. You don't have to do. You just allow yourself to be.

You could ask yourself:

What am I fearful about? Angry about? Sad about, etc.

Can you see how important it is to be congruent with your values and beliefs and how your life is affected if you are not?

Can you see how every repeated pattern/habit in your life can be attributed to your belief system?

Living your values and beliefs, being curious, reminding yourself every day of the life you want to live by embracing what you have discovered, and unapologetically living this way will help you to create the life you want very quickly.

My advice? Be passionate and 100% committed to your discoveries.

For those of you who would like a few more discoveries, here are some more sentences for you. Complete these in the same way, with no overthinking.

PART TWO
YOUR HISTORY OF DEVELOPMENT

If I try hard, then...

Life is about...

Love is about...

If I'm responsible, then...

There are times when life...

People are...

My family is...

It takes... to be successful.

...is outside my control.

There is no such thing as...

My friends are...

My Mum is...

My Dad is...

I am stressed when...

MENOPAUSE MIND SHIFTS

I am scared when…

I fear…

I want…

Cherish your discoveries. Write your own story. Design your own life and do it with love for yourself and your impact on this beautiful world.

If you struggle with any of this and would like some guidance, please feel free to email me. I would love to hear from you.

PART TWO
YOUR HISTORY OF DEVELOPMENT

Step 4: Speak Your Truth

This is one of my favourite things to talk about and encourage women to do. I'm not encouraging speaking badly or speaking in order to hurt someone, of course. Not that at all.

Your truth, in other words, your language. The words you choose to use are a force to be reckoned with. I know when I have something to say, and it is my absolute truth spoken from my core, then not only do I feel completely free to speak it, but I also don't mind if nobody agrees. It is my truth spoken from my soul from love and kindness. Never to hurt anyone.

We create our lives by either speaking our truth or denying ourselves of it. This, in turn, creates our emotional responses. Have you ever said yes when really you meant no? Maybe my question should actually be, how often have you said yes when you wanted to say no? In doing so, how often have you denied yourself peace and stillness within? How often have you created dis-ease within your body?

It's a double-edged sword to be true to yourself at the risk of hurting others. Yet, you cannot control other responses to your truth. You can, however, lead the way in demonstrating how they could also speak theirs.

I have absolute respect for the straight-talkers of this world. I know exactly where I am with them. I know that what they say is what they mean. I don't have to try to interpret anything and get it wrong. Misunderstandings happen all the time and can lead to the breakdown of many a good relationship.

When I was growing up, my dad was a yes man. He said yes all the time and then constantly let people down. As his children, this affected us immensely. How could we trust him? My Dad is the nicest person you will ever meet. His ability to say 'no' did not and does not exist for him. Why? He doesn't want to let anyone down. He wants to help

PART TWO
YOUR HISTORY OF DEVELOPMENT

everyone. He doesn't like confrontation in any form. It takes a lot more energy to understand what he actually means and wants. Over the years, that has been very difficult to manage emotionally. I can see over the years how I have taken on his behaviour. How detrimental it has been to my life. It was a relief to learn and let go. To release any expectations of him. To just love him for who he is. To see that his behaviour also comes from his own childhood adversity.

We hold so much power in what we say. Do we even realise this? I don't think so. Imagine what we might say in anger that then lingers in the mind of the recipient and grows bigger and bolder over time, affecting their behaviour. Now, imagine how we talk to ourselves. How easily we create drama within with the words in our heads and how this can have a catastrophic physical effect on our bodies.

How we speak to ourselves and allow others to speak to us all creates a chemical imbalance inside our bodies. How do you free yourself when a negative reaction occurs inside of you? Learn to speak your own truth with confidence and conviction. Stop allowing drama to consume you. Stop the expectations you have of others. Learn who you really are and want to be. Lead your life with absolute unconditional love.

Speaking your truth takes courage to start with. Like anything else, the more you practice, the easier it becomes. You are re-training yourself and showing those around you how you want to be treated.

This is what I would like you to try. Whenever you are going to say yes, and you FEEL a little niggle physically in your body, I want you to pause. Are you about to speak your truth? If that niggle is saying 'no,' that is precisely what I want you to say.

'No, not today, thank you'.

'No, that's not for me, thank you.'

PART TWO
YOUR HISTORY OF DEVELOPMENT

'No, I'm not available today; thanks for asking, though.'

'No, that's not something I am interested in, thank you.'

Sometimes, it is easier to have a few phrases up your sleeve. Good luck

Yes, it takes courage, but I know you have that inside of you. I just know you do. xx

Step 5: How does this affect your menopause journey?

Phew!!

All that we have discussed above, when known, re-written positively, and lived, will have such a transformational effect on your life and those around you. As our bodies age and menopause hormones take charge, whatever we can do to release tension held in our bodies can only have a positive, nurturing, and enhancing effect.

Our ability to cope with life events and stresses reduces during menopause, yet what I have found to be of great relief is understanding myself and what I want out of my life—understanding the limiting beliefs stuck inside, understanding which values were not being lived, being aware when I was not speaking my own truth and how that created such physical illness within me. My behaviour was ruled by old, outdated belief patterns, which kept

PART TWO
YOUR HISTORY OF DEVELOPMENT

cortisol levels too high and in a chronic state of leadership.

Discovering your values and beliefs and speaking your truth are the foundation of taking control of your menopause journey.

PART THREE
CONNECTION

There was a significant reason why I called my business 'Soul Decisions', and it had to do with connection. I imagined being with my clients and asking myself what was the deepest, most profound way that I could be alongside them on their journey to discovering who they truly are and want to be in life. I imagined my soul connecting with theirs, and it felt perfect.

I'm not a 'yes, I quite like that kind of girl; I'm more a 'I bloody love that, it's amazing!'

PART THREE
CONNECTION

If I am going to connect with you, we will be doing so on a soul level, filled with love and appreciation for you as another human being, and we will have a great time together. You are my inspiration, and I aim to be yours.

Now, I don't see people approaching life this way. I see busy, busy, busy, and I see disconnection.

I have done loads of self-development work and training, which connected me to all parts of myself and my life, yet there was always an element missing. What was that?

Decades worth of pain hidden in my heart and soul. Stealing my energy and vitality. Stealing my health. Stealing my ability to live with peace within. Stealing my ability to live with the core of who I am and my awareness of what I want for my life. The pain I was unable to access on a conscious level was screaming for connection and release. I did not know this.

Where do we find this release?

We find it in all the simple, effortless ways we connect to ourselves and life when we give ourselves permission and space when we breathe slowly and deeply. When we look into each other's eyes with love and appreciation. When we look around us in everyday life.

Here is an example of a text I sent to a friend on the other side of the world:

"I'm walking along the canal that runs near our new home. It is the most beautiful day. The sky is a vibrant blue, the sun is shining, and I can hear sheep in the field nearby and a tractor making its way through the next field. The air is crisp, cold, and refreshing as I slowly breathe in and out. I'm aware of the heat of my breath circulating the cold air and remember my kids always being fascinated with the sight of the misty cloud that comes from your mouth on beautiful days like these. I'm reminiscing about our connection to the teachings of the Maori culture

PART THREE
CONNECTION

from our years living in New Zealand and how it has truly inspired and enriched my life. I am acutely aware of my connection to my land, my river, my mountain, and my people, and I know I am home. My heart and soul are full in this moment xx.

What is genuine connection? The connection that means I can touch you, look into your eyes, hug you, be with you and not have to speak. I can sense your presence, hear your words, and see you for your wholeness. This type of connection is authentic and effortless.

The brilliance of technology has taken over the world, and we are now and have been for a long time, connecting on a vastly different level. The pandemic changed so much for humankind. 'Unprecedented times' was something seen frequently written and spoken on social media. Instead of talking face to face, it has become so easy to experience our family, friends, colleagues, and strangers through words or visions we see on a screen of some kind. Technology has opened a pandora's box of communication that has now become a way of life, and in doing so, are we losing the essence of connection? Maybe, maybe not?

Without technology, I could not have sent an 'in the moment' message to my friend in New Zealand at a time when she was sleeping.

We look externally of ourselves at what is not working. We read books, attend seminars, and sign up for different courses, all of which are great to a point. We search for how to overcome things, how to re-frame things, searching for the next big something that will show us how to feel better about ourselves and our lives. All of these things do make us feel better and allow us to see our worlds differently. They can put an extra spring in our steps for sure. But what is actually happening? What is still missing?

The answer to these very valuable questions is:

PART THREE
CONNECTION

'We are disconnected from ourselves at our core,' and we don't even realise it most of the time.'

We aren't dealing with the core of why we self-sabotage, feel lonely, sad, anxious, procrastinate, and feel lost. Why are we so disconnected from ourselves? It is too painful to go there, and each time we do, we re-traumatise ourselves.

Our nervous systems are on overdrive.

It once felt easy and natural to pick up the phone for a chat or to visit someone at home. These days, it's so easy to send a quick text while doing something else. The tempo has picked up. Multitasking is considered acceptable, so the race is on to fit more in. We fill schedules for our kids with 4 or 5 activities a week, as well as school and homework. How do they learn about downtime and the importance of it? Don't get me wrong; I love to live life fully. The busyness of life has taken over for most people, and we have lost the beautiful, slow side of connection. Being with someone physically and being totally present in that moment and being with ourselves in silence and stillness. Yet what do we crave?

I feel so passionate about this one word, 'connection,' and the meaning and connotations it has for us as a human race. I want to explore connection as we navigate menopause. What does it mean to you? Have you even thought of its importance? What it means to you to stay connected to yourself, each other, to your land, your river, your mountain, this moment.

Your inner Connection
Take a slow, deep breath.

Take a slow, deep breath, and as you breathe out, allow your shoulders to drop.

Take a slow, deep breath and scan your body. For each part you feel tension, breathe again, focus on that area, and with intention, allow it to feel heavy, soft, and relaxed.

PART THREE
CONNECTION

Breathing slowly, gently close your eyes....and look……. what do you see?

Put this book down, and for a few more minutes, just be with this beautiful moment.

Nothing to do. Nowhere to go.

Just be.

A vast world of possibilities awaits you when you have a genuine connection with yourself. Connection with who you are and who you want to be, and then there is the world that surrounds you. Your world, your environment. The one you have created for yourself. Your immediate world of people and places, thoughts, and dreams. The bigger world, the universe, goes beyond that. The amazing vast expansion of you lies within it all, and you are connected to it all, and we are connected to each other.

How amazing.

When I say the word connection, I feel it in my heart and soul. Our modern world, I feel, has both created connection and harmed connection.

What is connection for you?

For me, it is truly being with myself. Connecting with my core values and beliefs. Loving who I am and the contribution I bring to this beautiful planet. Knowing that I have so much love to give and giving it freely. It is being with and contributing to the lives of others. It is loving unconditionally. Being completely present in the now of every moment. Showing myself and others love and compassion.

I have come to realise that without connection, life takes on dull tones. The dance of life becomes empty and lonely. Isolation takes hold, and hiding away becomes a way of life. We enter a world of our own where the energy and vitality of the human spirit are barely felt. For some of us, this isolation is the life to which we become accustomed without realising it. An isolated life without connection is a

PART THREE
CONNECTION

life that squashes our confidence, challenges our resilience, and questions our identity and purpose in this lifetime. We weave in and out of each day without clarity of purpose for the day ahead, and we repeat this over and over again.

If we are lucky, one day, we will wake up!

When menopause had me in a tight grip, I was unable to connect. I hid myself away for days. Unable to give, barely able to speak, to plan, to process what was going on in my head. The feeling of going mad, out of control, was so real and so exhausting. I couldn't get to grips with what was going on. Some days, I felt like my spirit was dying away. I stopped connecting with friends and could barely connect with people I loved. Worst of all, I couldn't connect with my son, who, like me, is a high-spirited, full of life, enthusiastic, strong character. His character became too much for me to bear. I wanted and needed to shut down, find peace and stillness, and, most of all, remain there while I tried to figure this whole menopause thing out. <u>I had no energy to do that; figure it out!</u>

I now know there was nothing to figure out in that moment. Being OK with the stillness inside myself would have been enough if I had known then what I know now. If I had been able to access the stillness as I can now.

I once heard someone say:

> *'You already have within you*
> *the ability to cope with any*
> *situation. Know that you have*
> *been given the obstacle you have*
> *been given because the solution*
> *already resides within you!'*

Mmmmm, it was not something I believed at the time, but something I allowed myself to be curious about. So here is what I think and believe now.

The statement is true. I think it is genius to be told that everything you need is already within you.

PART THREE
CONNECTION

Your job is to be still enough to see the answer when it is revealed and the courage to step forward. If you continue to rush around, you will not see what is always laid before you—the gift in the moment.

What has happened to us over time is that we have lost connection with our intuition. The fast pace of life and expectations of ourselves and others prevent us from experiencing the stillness in which our intuition lies. I see it every day in all walks of life. We become unaware of ourselves. In order to become aware, we need to connect to the stillness that is within us all. Meditation, journaling, and sharing our innermost thoughts and feelings with someone we trust will all reveal areas we feel stuck in our lives and answers to many internal questions. Your intuition is never wrong. It will always guide you in the right direction. Guide you towards your own growth and way of being in this world. All you need to do is tune in to you. Connect fully with yourself.

How?

By paying attention to your instincts, hunches, your physical body, your feelings and being still long enough to connect with what you are intuitively telling yourself.

During my menopause journey, I have certainly felt like I was spinning out of control. I forgot that stillness was possible. In fact, I am not sure I even considered it to be a thing. What I knew was that peace and being peaceful was foreign to me. Not possible for me. Not even something I was aware I was searching desperately for. I was searching so hard for something that I thought would never come, and I didn't know what that was. I was a bit of a mess inwardly. I was completely disconnected, not trusting myself. I know that some of you can relate to this. My clients have all struggled with the same or similar.

Connection to our true selves is something so achievable, and as humans, we are born for

PART THREE
CONNECTION

connection, biologically wired for it. We can transform our lives when we let go of limiting beliefs and the high expectations we have of ourselves. We can discover who we truly are at our core— discovering our true values and speaking our own truth. Acting and reacting according to what is true to us is very empowering.

When you can do this, your authenticity will shine through impacting your relationships and how you connect with your family, friends, colleagues, and strangers. Your outlook on life will improve tenfold. Your world will internally and externally become a better place. Your true potential will unfold.

All of this is achievable when you reveal what is at your core to release the pain held there, and this can only be done through experience and connection with others to help you.

PART FOUR
YOUR COACHING
JOURNEY

I love Life Coaching. It is such a positive way to go on a journey of self-discovery and get results quickly. It is even better when you find yourself an outstanding Coach to work with. Okay, I am slightly biased, but also not. It is great to do both. That is to read and discover things for yourself and find someone who will be able to see the things you cannot and share, softly challenge those things with you. It can also be an emotional journey, so sharing

PART FOUR
YOUR COACHING JOURNEY

that with someone you trust is invaluable and life-transforming.

In the following pages, allow your imagination to run free. Allow all that you desire to reveal itself and show you the life you want to be living and that which you want to let go of. The following coaching journey and the previous discovery chapters on values and beliefs are all setting the foundations of the life you want to lead in a way that is congruent with who you want to be in this lifetime.

To discover this lifestyle, we need to see what is out of alignment. We know what it is like to be out of alignment in our bodies because we feel it, so as you go through each exercise, be present to what you feel and where you feel it in your body and again allow it just to be.

As you go through your menopause journey, what do you want from your life?

MENOPAUSE MIND SHIFTS

Make a list of all the things you want in your life. Then, continue with the following exercises.

PART FOUR
YOUR COACHING JOURNEY

Step 6: Discovering Your Ideal Self

Each of us has an ideal self that we would like to be. Let's get some clarity on who you would like to be, what you want out of your life and what is missing.

Your **surface self** goes about living day to day without questioning her experiences.

Your **core self** wants to break free and live a fulfilling life filled with meaningful experiences.

Ideal Average Day: The day that, if you were to live it every day, would always be healthy for you, sustainable, and you'd love to experience.

If you were living your Ideal Average Day every day…

o   Where would you live?
o   What would your house look like?

MENOPAUSE MIND SHIFTS

- What is the view like?
- What would you have for breakfast?
- Who are you with?
- What do you talk about?
- What does the mundane stuff in life look like?
- What would you spend your mornings doing?
- What about the afternoons?
- What would you do for lunch? Who are you with? What's the conversation?
- Who are your friends?
- How do you spend your time with them?
- How does this make you feel?
- What do you talk about?
- What do you do that is purposeful?
- What do you do for personal fulfilment?
- What do you have for dinner?
- What time do you go to bed, and what is your routine?

Some wider questions:

- What are you striving for?

PART FOUR
YOUR COACHING JOURNEY

- What is important to you? Break this down into the details of what and why.
- What adventures do you want to have?
- What legacy will you leave?
- What is missing from your life?

Spend some time exploring what these questions provoke in you and what you realise about your life and how you want to live.

One of the main questions I ask my clients:

What do you want for your life?

It is profoundly surprising how many people don't stop to ask themselves this question on a deeper level than instant gratification. Only if you know what you want your life to be like and then make decisions based on the answer will you either begin to live the life you want or create the life you want by design.

MENOPAUSE MIND SHIFTS

Now that you have some idea of what you want, write more to discover why you want it.

.

PART FOUR
YOUR COACHING JOURNEY

Step 7: Overcoming Fear

How do we overcome fear during menopause when our chemical imbalance is a contributing factor? Well, the more we feel the fear, the more we increase that chemical imbalance. Over the edge we go.

Fear is there when we think about our challenges. The more we think about the challenge, the more it grows; the more we think about it, the more it grows. We have given it the focus it does not deserve, and as we do that, we get more of it. The more focused, the more it magnifies. The more it magnifies, the more intense the feelings and thoughts are, and we are trapped. Trapped focusing on something we do like or want in our lives. It's a never-ending loop. Round and round we go. Year after year. That is, until we identify what is happening in order to let it go or we learn techniques that allow us to let it go without question. Sometimes, we don't want to let go. There is a familiar comfort to our discomfort. How crazy we are! How complex we can be. Easier to say that now I have strategies and tools in place that allow me to let go quickly and easily. That was not how it once was. How torturous life was when I had a meaning for everything, usually making it all about me, paralysed with destructive thoughts and emotions, all based in fear. Reacting in my life from a place of fear.

How did I know this? Let's explore:

Symptoms that will tell you you're on the wheel of fear...

- Constant impatience, desire for instant answers for instant relief from the tension of not knowing.
- Ongoing exhaustion where everything seems to be too much effort.
- Racing around, but nothing gets done.
- Self-righteousness where everyone else has the problem.
- You're underappreciated.

PART FOUR
YOUR COACHING JOURNEY

- You're constantly misunderstood, and people keep taking you the wrong way.
- A paranoia that you never get enough support.
- Numbness in your feelings and thoughts, and you deny anything is wrong.
- Guilt and shame – everything is your fault.
- Out of control.
- Wasting time.
- Easily overwhelmed and bogged down.
- You feel singled out for getting it wrong, and no one understands how hard it is for you.
- You believe you're alone feeling that way, and there's nothing that can be done by you.

What can you relate to?

Mmmmm, next questions:

- If you knew you could handle whatever life had to offer, what would you attempt or endeavour to do?
- Are you doing it?

- If you didn't worry, what would you endeavour to do?
- Are you doing it?
- What would you focus on instead?
- What would you think about instead?
- What would you start to do?
- What would you stop doing?
- What would you explore?

Courage turns up when we take action. We take action even when we don't feel like it. The thing that then challenged us is no longer of concern. We are ready for our next level of growth.

Fear-based excuses.

We have our go-to excuses when fear presents itself to us. Things like:

- 'I haven't got time.'
- 'I'm too busy.'
- 'It's not the right time.'
- 'I have to do this with the kids.'

PART FOUR
YOUR COACHING JOURNEY

What are yours?

Language choices

Here are some language options to help you out of the fear cycle:

- Your language becomes your experience.
- Your language determines your experience.

Change your language, and you change your perception of your experience.

I can't...	Choose **'I won't.'**
I should...	Choose **'I could.'**
It's a problem...	Choose **'It's an opportunity.'**
I hope...	Choose **'I wonder.'**
I wish...	Choose **'I wonder.'**
What if...	Choose **'Maybe'**

MENOPAUSE MIND SHIFTS

Which of these fear-based emotions do you relate to?

Anger	Shame
Impatience	Guilt
Exhaustion	Defeated
Self-Righteousness	Out of control
Misunderstood	Confused
Paranoid	Overwhelmed
Paralysed	Victimised

You don't have to feel any of these emotions. They all relate to something you are telling yourself. They relate to something you are convincing yourself of. They all relate to you not having full responsibility for your life. Here is where you show yourself compassion. Love yourself through the realisation of why these emotions exist and realise that being

PART FOUR
YOUR COACHING JOURNEY

stuck here is a total waste of your time and vibrant life.

When I reflect on those difficult years, I can honestly say I felt all the above. All of them. I was silently fighting to get out of feeling any of them when I knew, in reality, I had so much joy in my life. An amazing husband, two gorgeous, well-grounded kids, a lovely home by the beach, fabulous friends, and a great job. What the heck was going on?

Pick the word from the list below that gives you the most intense reaction when you put it in the following sentence...

"If someone I love, respect, and admire were to think I was…................., I'd be devastated."

Intense reaction words:

- Selfish
- A loser
- Stupid

- A fake
- Weak
- Lazy
- Incompetent
- Invisible
- Ordinary
- Rejected

When you know what you're most afraid of, you're better prepared to create a proactive choice and response rather than a knee-jerk reaction.

The more I learned about myself and the more I learned strategies to help me calm my nervous system during menopause, the better I felt. I no longer cared about the word that went into that sentence above. I no longer carried the crippling level of emotional fear from the list above.

All of it came from a time that no longer existed, and I was no longer the person it belonged to back then. I had grown. Grown and was able to shed what was holding me hostage and fueling my menopause

PART FOUR
YOUR COACHING JOURNEY

symptoms. Ascension meditation was the catalyst for letting go and living with so much more peace and true joy in my life. It opened my eyes and released my heart.

I love it so much that I have dedicated an entire chapter for you later in the book.

For now, I trust that this exercise has helped you to realise where fear is holding you hostage. As we go through the following exercises, we will unravel more of who you are, who you want to be and the kind of life you want to live.

Remember love and compassion for yourself. Always.

Step 8: Becoming Selfish

I love this section of the coaching journey because it has always brought up the response of 'I couldn't possibly' or 'oooooh no!' when I ask what the word selfish means to them.

Often misunderstood. Especially, I find, by women. Selfish is a word that can bring up some interesting 'stuff.' For sure.

- Are you governed by what others want and expect of you, and you couldn't possibly think of yourself and your own needs first?
- Are you a prisoner to outside expectations?
- Where do your dreams, desires, needs, and wants fit into your world?

Many women go through years of always putting others first. We all do it for different reasons. A classic example is if you have kids. Demanding little creatures' kids (I'm smiling, by the way), I distinctly remember thinking to myself and saying to my husband that I would give the kids what I didn't have. I was determined to look back on their childhood with no regrets. No regrets about missing out on anything, and to the best of my ability, I stuck to it. No problem at all until menopause came crashing into my life and robbed my energy. Luckily, though, they had a solid foundation from which to experience their mother. Thank goodness. At least, I think they had. We might have to ask them! I might have been crazy all along and didn't realise it!

So, when you see the word selfish, what does it conjure up for you? What is your first response?

Here are some questions to get you thinking:

- Who runs your life?
- Do you want to be liked?
- Do you worry that if you don't 'go along,' you won't belong?
- Do you sacrifice, unconsciously, your hopes and dreams to keep others placated?

- Do you know how to say 'no' to others and 'yes' to yourself?
- Do you speak your truth?

There is a difference between being selfish and being needy.

Selfish – you put your needs first. You value yourself, your opinions, your actions, your choices, your life, and all of this is OK and good for your health. This is my positive definition of selfish. So, a certain amount of selfishness is essential. There is so much value in this positive side to selfishness, both for you and what you are teaching others. You are looking after yourself. There is absolutely nothing wrong with that. Nothing at all.

The ugly side of selfishness is described in the dictionary alongside words like egotistical, greedy, narcissist, self-centred, etc. This is not what I am talking about here. This way of being is not very attractive at all, not easy to live with and comes from fear.

PART FOUR
YOUR COACHING JOURNEY

Being 'Needy'. Now, this is a different kettle of fish, so to speak. I used to listen to everyone's problems. Always there, going above and beyond. Taking over situations because I thought I could handle them better and knew all the answers. I filled my boots with being indispensable in all aspects of my life. This started from a very early age.

'I'm sitting on the sofa, and it's time to go back. My heart feels like it is ripping out of my chest, and I am screaming inside.

So much pain all the time. It's exhausting. I feel frantic and desperate, clinging on to every minute.

I don't want to go back. In my head, I am screaming, 'Don't make me go back' as our things are packed yet again into carrier bags, ready for the trip.

In this moment, I just want to die. I want this leaving and not knowing to finally stop. Death, I feel, would put a silence to it all.

I somehow manage to say, 'If I go back there, I am going to commit suicide.'

I'm ten years old.

Now, it takes a desperate child to mean these words, and I was desperate. When I sat on the sofa at my dad's house that day, I knew I wasn't going back to live with Mum and my sisters. I didn't have the relationship with my mum that they had. Or that is what I believed at the time. I didn't know where I belonged anymore.

My Dad was everything to me. Everything. I was totally lost without him in my life when I was little. The void that was created when he disappeared could not be filled even though I tried.

I created and mastered the need to be needed.

To fit in with my Dad and Step mum, I created and mastered the need to be needed and acted in a

PART FOUR
YOUR COACHING JOURNEY

way to be helpful in many aspects of my life. Not to be a burden. I did what was needed in gratitude for having a roof over my head and food on the table. I figured out how to fit into this other family my Dad now had. I found a way to belong until I couldn't do it anymore. Everything came crashing down, and one day, I did not belong anywhere. Mum was with my sisters, and I had distanced myself so much I couldn't go back. Dad was with his other family, and I could no longer conform. I spent years perfecting my role of being needed only to find it was not sustainable, nor was it easing the sadness that engulfed me. In some ways, though, it gave me significance at a time in my life when I was needy of some love and attention, and I would get that from the people whose problems I was able to solve.

It's quite exhausting when you create this persona that people cannot do without you. Many women do this to their detriment. Then menopause comes along, and bam! We can't do it anymore. Unfortunately, at this stage in life, we have set the scene by which people know us, depend on us, and, therefore, treat us. When this happens, asking for help is very difficult, and people around us don't always know how to help. So, it is time to become positively selfish for the sake of our own health and wellness.

It's up to everyone to meet their own needs, and being selfish in a positive way helps you to do this. It is a good thing to pass on to our children. I am going to say here, especially our girls. We are, after all, still in a male-dominated world.

Here are some more things for you to think about:

How could you put yourself first and be OK with it? Where would you start that would make a difference in your life?

As Einstein put it, *"The sign of insanity is doing the same thing over and over again and expecting a different result."*

PART FOUR
YOUR COACHING JOURNEY

Put your desires first (gasp!)

As you become more comfortable with being selfish, you will gain more confidence and strength. This may shake relationships a little at first. Don't worry about that. Your behaviour will rub off, you will gain more respect, and you will attract others who are comfortable with a strong person.

You will need less from others. They will require less from you. You will feel more independent and less reliant on what others think of you, as well as becoming more generous in a healthy way as you have more to give.

What is the 'thing' you've dreamed of that you've been putting off?

For you to grow, you need to be selfish – you need to be willing to take care of your needs and to prioritise them – as in, put them in your diary, set aside the time, focus on them, nurture them and care about them.

Questions

What will it take for you to pay attention to the call of your heart rather than pay attention to what others want of you?

Do you have a vision of yourself that is greater than what others see you as?

Can you accept that it's reasonable to put your needs first?

What is something you could say 'yes' to that would make YOU happy?

What if you didn't mind not 'keeping the peace'?

What if you were OK with a little 'rocking the boat'?

The next important thing:

Get clear on who you spend your time with.

PART FOUR
YOUR COACHING JOURNEY

- Is it people who expect you to stay the same and never change or grow?
- Is it people who celebrate or belittle your successes?
- Is it people who pursue dreams, or are 'dream' snatchers?

It's daring to pursue your passions, interests, wants, and needs and sometimes actually doing something for you before you do something for someone else.

Tips:

Instead of saying 'yes' because you don't want to say 'no,' say – 'Can I get back to you?' and give yourself some space to consider the request calmly.

Become aware of those habits within you that volunteer your time and skills at the expense of your energy and health.

MENOPAUSE MIND SHIFTS

Instead of saying 'yes,' say 'I will, but first I want to...' and put your desires first.

What is it you desire?

PART FOUR
YOUR COACHING JOURNEY

Step 9: Developing Generosity

Why this chapter? Didn't I tell you to become selfish in the last chapter, and now I'm confusing you? Aren't we over-generous usually as women anyway, running around after everyone else? Over giving. Overstretching ourselves.

I Googled and found the seven forms of generosity: thoughts, words, money, time, things, influence, and attention.

What do you show yourself, ladies?

Generosity is described as:

'Involves giving to others not simply anything in abundance but rather giving those things that are good for others. Generosity always intends to enhance the true well-being of those to whom it gives.'

'Generous people are those who give more than what is expected of them.'

Well, yes, this is the majority of women I know.

In the Life Coaching world and influenced by the work of Tony Robbins, we talk about the six core needs of the human race. These are:

- Certainty: The need to feel safe and secure.
- Variety: The need for novelty and excitement.
- Significance: The need to feel important and valued.
- Connection/Love: The need to feel loved and connected to others.
- Growth: The need to learn and develop.
- Contribution: The need to make a difference in the world.

How generous are you with yourself in relation to these needs?

Here are some specific ways in which generosity can meet our six core needs:

PART FOUR
YOUR COACHING JOURNEY

Certainty: When we help others, it can give us a sense of control and predictability in our lives. We know that we are making a difference, and that can help us feel more secure.

Variety: Helping others can give us a new perspective on life and introduce us to new people and experiences. This can help us break out of our comfort zones and feel more alive.

Significance: When we help others, we are making a statement about our values and our worth. We are showing that we care about others and that we want to make a difference in the world. This can give us a sense of purpose and meaning.

Connection/Love: Helping others is a great way to connect with others and build relationships. It shows that we care about others and that we are willing to put their needs before our own. This can help us feel loved and supported.

Growth: Helping others can challenge us to grow and develop as individuals. It can teach us new skills, help us learn about different cultures, and make us more compassionate and understanding.

Contribution: Helping others is a way of contributing to the world and making it a better place. It can give us a sense of satisfaction and fulfilment, knowing that we are making a difference.

Contribution is where I feel developing generosity fits in. As we age, our ability to contribute to something bigger than ourselves seems more important. It gives you a feeling of fulfilment when you contribute something of yourself. When your generous contribution is more expansive than your close family and friends or even the job you choose. When you add value because you enjoy it (and this is key: you enjoy it), people are naturally attracted to you, and you fill your body with the right chemicals to feed your soul.

PART FOUR
YOUR COACHING JOURNEY

It's a mature soul that gives generously because it feels great. No attachments. No expectations.

Something to pay attention to.

The potential downsides of generosity in relation to the six core needs:

Certainty: When we are constantly giving to others, it can be easy to lose sight of our own needs and feel insecure about our own future. We may worry that we will not have enough for ourselves or that we will not be able to meet our own needs.

Variety: When we are constantly giving to others, it can be easy to get stuck in a rut and feel like we are not living a fulfilling life. We may miss out on new experiences and opportunities because we are always putting others first.

Significance: When we are not careful, generosity can become a way of seeking validation from others. We may give in order to feel important or loved rather than because we genuinely want to help. This can lead to feelings of resentment and burnout.

Connection/Love: When we are constantly giving to others, it can be easy to neglect our own relationships. We may not have time for our loved ones, or we may not be able to give them the attention they need. This can lead to feelings of isolation and loneliness.

Growth: When we are constantly giving to others, it can be easy to stop growing and developing as individuals. We may not have time for self-care (very important, please pay attention) or for learning new things. This can lead to feelings of stagnation and boredom.

Contribution: When we are not careful, generosity can become a way of avoiding our own problems. We may give in order to feel better about ourselves rather than because we truly want to help others. This can lead to feelings of guilt and

PART FOUR
YOUR COACHING JOURNEY

inadequacy, being overwhelmed or being taken for granted.

It is essential to be aware of these potential downsides so that we can avoid them. If we are generous in a way that is healthy and sustainable, it can be a wonderful way to meet our six core needs. However, if we are not careful, it can also lead to negative consequences.

Here are some tips for being a generous person without neglecting your own needs:

Give freely and without expectations. Don't give in order to get something in return. Give because you want to help others and because it makes you feel good.

Set boundaries. Decide how much time and money you are willing to give and stick to it. Don't feel guilty about saying no to requests that you can't or don't want to fulfil.

MENOPAUSE MIND SHIFTS

Take care of yourself. Make sure to get enough sleep, eat healthy foods, and exercise regularly. Take time for yourself to relax and de-stress.

Find a balance. Don't give so much that you neglect your own needs. Find a balance between giving to others and taking care of yourself.

On the flip side, if someone gives and then feels depleted, they did it to 'get' something in return. Was it the need for significance? For love? For certainty? To prove how lovely or kind you are? Please pay attention here. Do you over give? If you do, what are you feeding within yourself? What is missing in your life, or what are you trying to prove? This area that needs attention can be very subtle and a blind spot for many women.

If you feel depleted when you are giving, ask yourself why. Ask yourself if you really want to do it.

Give without thought of what will come back and do it because it feels good for you, nothing else. Not

PART FOUR
YOUR COACHING JOURNEY

because you feel guilty or obliged. So many women feel obliged to do things or guilt-ridden if they don't. These actions weigh heavy on our souls. They fuel the already stressed hormonal imbalance in our bodies as we menopause. They are usually acted out for the wrong reasons and never feel good.

All you have to do is tune into your body. It will tell you if something is right or wrong. Your intuition will tell you. Just pay attention.

Don't seduce or manipulate – having the attitude of, 'I did this, so you must do that...' No one owes you anything. Really, nobody owes you anything. Is there a secret part of you that may feel this unknowingly?

When you give from a place of peace within yourself, your creativity will flow, and you will feel energised and joyful. There does not need to be any focus put on being taken for granted, appreciated or the expectation of reciprocity.

Questions for your consideration:

What do the people close to you value, and how do you know this?

What gives you joy? Is it intellectual pursuits? Creative pursuits?

What about your passions would others want to know about – as long as they share the passion?

Where are others providing value to you? i.e., acts of kindness, going out of their way for you, taking care of things for you, volunteering for things that take time, being kind when you're not kind.

Are you unreasonable about what you expect of others? Do you get dramatic if others don't pay attention to your 'needs'?

If no one is paying you attention, how do you feel?

PART FOUR
YOUR COACHING JOURNEY

Get clear on the following:

Do you give to others to 'get something at some time?

Do you NOT do something for someone because they didn't do something for you?

Do you engage in silent payback – where the other person has no idea they crossed you?

Do others have to acknowledge your value? So, if you are spiritual, do others have to know this and even agree with it for you to feel useful? – This is hostage-taking.

Try to:

Be OK with giving without the need for it to be appreciated, validated, noticed, or mentioned.

Provide value to others to improve their lives, not your own.

Give when people aren't watching, and don't tell anyone.

Don't draw attention to what you give.

This section is intended to help you consider your life from a different perspective. To discover some blind spots. To question some behaviours that may be keeping you stuck in old patterns that no longer serve you.

After reading this section, is there anything about your life that you would want to change?

PART FOUR
YOUR COACHING JOURNEY

Step 10: Embracing Uncertainty

Many people fall short of dreams and goals or don't even attempt them because they would rather stay comfortable with their 'comfort zone.'

Yet 'All progress takes place OUTSIDE your comfort zone.' A fundamental aspect of life is growth. Your growth. To grow, we must embrace uncertainty.

Do you:

- shut down.
- have low energy.
- live in fear.
- withdraw.
- say, it's not important anymore.
- give up.
- stay in a 'rut.'
- criticise people who have a go.

MENOPAUSE MIND SHIFTS

Your ability and willingness to live at cause and to take 100% responsibility for your results and non-results will assist with this.

PART FIVE
LETTER TO THE KIDS

Being a parent is not easy. You have the responsibility of influencing the life of another human being, and to be honest, we don't always get it right. When I was at my least functioning, when the days dragged from one to the next, I could barely get my head off the pillow. I would walk around the house feeling the weight of everything that needed to be done to help maintain some form of normality in our home. It took me every ounce of energy to keep up appearances, especially for the

PART FIVE
LETTER TO THE KIDS

kids. I felt heartbroken, lost in my own private, vulnerable world of menopause symptoms.

As a parent, I had been determined to raise my children very differently from how I was raised. My relationship with them to be solid, safe, secure, and filled with unconditional love. No matter what. To show them love always. During those very dark days of early menopause, when I struggled immensely to keep myself together, my childhood losses came back to haunt me. The unspoken promises I made to myself about what kind of mother I would be were challenged to the core. At times, I had nothing to give them. As teenagers, they struggled with their hormones; I was struggling with mine at the other end of the scale.

I know I wasn't alone in this. I know many of you feel the same.

At this time, I said things I would never normally have said. I could not cope with the stress of anger outbursts or any form of disagreement or drama that entered our home. I know that I repressed their feelings; I overreacted at times. I was right. They were wrong, and they must listen to me. No longer able to give them space to express themselves easily. My most precious young humans were suffering, especially my strong-willed amazing boy who was experiencing hormone surges himself more than my gentle-natured beautiful daughter.

He would express intense anger, which always seemed aimed at me. We certainly have the same strength of character. I have always loved his zest for life, high energy, and passion for everything he does. His outward, robust, delightful approach to inventing or sports was infectious and inspirational. When menopause hit, I couldn't keep up with the high energy. What ensued was a battle of I was right, and he had to listen to me. He was right, and I had to listen to him as he got louder and louder to prove his point. Or more frustrated with me because somehow, I had changed. Neither of us understood what was going on. We couldn't reason out the

PART FIVE
LETTER TO THE KIDS

situation that inevitably turned into a full-scale shout-out, resulting in him slamming his bedroom door and raging around, throwing things inside his bedroom. Of course, I knew I was the adult and should have been much more emotionally together, but I just couldn't. I couldn't find the energy or the vocabulary to reason or even calm myself or the situation. I knew it, but I couldn't do anything about it at the time. My kids were used to being able to express themselves, and suddenly, I was no longer there even though I was physically there. No longer able to hold the space for them to express their emotions fully. I was trapped in this locked, suffocating box called menopause, and someone had thrown away the key.

As a mum, I wanted them both to grow and flourish. To live life to the full with joy and excitement. To know that they are loved unconditionally and, to embrace all opportunities, to give things a go. To fail, make mistakes and know that it's all OK because you are an amazing human,

You could ask yourself, what do you know now from the experience that you did not know before? How have you grown because of the experience? How has it shaped the person you are today?

We are here to grow, develop and constantly learn, which means making mistakes. It's from the mistakes that we usually learn our biggest lessons. It's from the hardship that we learn how genuinely resilient we are. When you share what you have learned about a situation, you will give others the gift of awareness for themselves. This is another important acknowledgement. Sharing your wisdom. Sharing your experience for someone else to understand from a different perspective. Something they have as a blind spot. We all have them. Curiosity is a key advantage in these situations. Being curious about different perspectives. It's so light and lovely being curious.

So, are you stuck? Do you believe that moments from the past are still in control of your life? This will

PART FIVE
LETTER TO THE KIDS

show itself when you repeatedly refer to past events negatively, not only in your language but also in how your body feels as you repeat the scenarios.

We have persistent illusions. The illusion that we are in control, yet really, we can only control ourselves. Can't we? I certainly have no control over how someone acts or reacts. Quite frankly, I don't want that responsibility either. My fight as a mum back then was to exercise what I thought was my right to control a situation and another human being. Stacey and Paul Martino call this 'Demand Parenting'. Yes, I tried that Demand Parenting thing!! Not very effective. I would not recommend it.

What about perceived failure? If you are still alive, how could you have possibly failed? How does this stop you from living? I could have constantly seen myself as failing as a mum when in an argument with my fantastic boy. I did fall into that trap of seeing myself as failing for a short time. It made me feel even worse. I wasn't showing myself any compassion at all. But I wasn't failing. I was having a really tough time, as many mums do.

If you are having a tough time, please know that does not equate to being a failure if that is what you are telling yourself. Choose to see all the good that you are. Choose to leave the past where it should be in the past. It's only an image. It is not present now in reality. It is imaginary. What's happening now is grief for what was, what could have been, and what should have been, and at some point, grief decides we cannot sit with this anymore. It is time to move on without blame.

So, ultimately, forgiveness is the gift you give to yourself to set yourself free.

'Dear Em and Matt

I don't know where to start or what will be written on this paper throughout this letter. I just know that

PART FIVE
LETTER TO THE KIDS

I want to try to explain and apologise for why I have behaved in such a weird way over the past months.

As we age, women experience this thing called menopause. It is a time in our lives when our worlds can be turned upside down. Mine has felt that way. Our bodies change so dramatically that we can lose who we are. I feel vulnerable and lost most days.

I know my behaviour has changed towards you. I know I have been more vacant and snappy, not really with you. I feel exhausted all the time. My body hurts and now feels so weak. I can't think straight, and I am haunted by experiences from my childhood that are filled with anxiety and fear. As I write this, I think, 'Isn't that strange for an adult to say?'

I have been so used to being in control and having lots of energy to do all sorts of things with you, but that is not the case at the moment.

MENOPAUSE MIND SHIFTS

I'm finding that I cannot cope with any kind of stress, and I'm struggling to concentrate when you want to tell me any of the things that are upsetting you.

I want you to know that I love you both so much. You are my world, and whatever I may have said, done or not done, that has hurt you, I am truly sorry.

Come and talk to me about whatever bothers you. We will just take it slowly and calmly.

One day, all of this will pass. I promise.

I love you both so much.

Mum

xx

PART SIX
ASCENSION
MEDITATION

"There is no need to look any further when you find the thing that works. Just keep doing it and let the magic unfold."

Soul Decisions Coaching

This, for me, was Ascension meditation. It was the first 'thing' that started to and continues to give

PART SIX
ASCENSION MEDITATION

me the gift and knowledge of living fully every moment of every day. Effortlessly.

So, let's first clear up a couple of misconceptions:

1) "I can't meditate because I can't clear my mind." You do not have to clear your mind of thoughts. Why? Well, because it is impossible to do so. The function of your mind is to keep you safe, to give you instruction, and to guide you through life...

2) "I can't meditate; I'm too stressed" Er, hello? Simply put, when we are stressed, our body floods with ugly chemicals, and we create a stress response that loops repeatedly within our bodies. We become hyper-sensitive in our reactions, which is consistently fuelled by the chemical reaction flowing through our system. Meditating allows our system to slow down, reducing the chemical reaction and calming our nervous system. In reality, we find ourselves less reactive, having better relationships, being less opinionated and judgmental, calmer, more grounded, and kinder to ourselves and others.

MENOPAUSE MIND SHIFTS

We see and feel more joy and happiness, love, and peace. The best bit…. the more you commit to meditating, the better it gets.

Imagine your daily life based and focused on praise, love, gratitude, and compassion. Many of us wander through life focused on fear, lack, scarcity, and judgment, seemingly unaware that we can change this if we pay attention and believe it is possible, even if we don't know how. As my beautiful friend Aditi says:

> *"When we believe change is possible, change happens."*
>
> Aditi Ishaya

Getting the most out of my life happened when I believed change was possible, and I learned the practice of Ascension. Until then, I had not believed change on such a deep level was possible. I wasn't even aware of the self-sabotaging, fear-based behaviours anymore, as they had just become a way

PART SIX
ASCENSION MEDITATION

of my being for so long. They had well and truly ingrained themselves into my everyday life.

Until one day.

One precious and wonderful day, I was so desperate that I decided to ask for help, and help came in the form of a movie.

As I sat watching the film 'A Mindful Choice,' I felt at peace for the first time in my entire life. Change WAS possible, and change WAS coming. I didn't know how; I just knew it was on its way because now I had a new, unique, and beautifully welcomed awareness that it was possible.

Shortly after watching A Mindful Choice, I embarked on a First Sphere training weekend. I was about to learn a technique that would change my life. ...

My next best decision was to commit 100%.

Committed 100% to *'Prioritising my peace.'* (You can try this; it is wonderful.)

…. So, in any situation I found myself in that would rock me into an unhealthy pattern of thinking or behaviour, I very quickly reminded myself to

'Prioritise my peace.'

Where is peace for you? Is peace only available when we sit cross-legged in meditation pose in the middle of a retreat or alone at the top of a mountain looking over a spectacular breathtaking view? What is your belief about this? I know I used to believe something like it.

Or is it possible to experience peace at any time, anywhere? Is it possible that it could be a state of being? I used to think constantly about taking myself away somewhere from all the hustle, bustle, and exhaustion of the life I was leading, especially the life that was going on in my head! Could someone just take me away from this? I felt squashed and

PART SIX
ASCENSION MEDITATION

beaten down. Until I discovered Ascension, it was a turning point in my life and significantly impacted my menopause journey. From the moment I learned the technique, I have been wholeheartedly 100% committed to daily practice. Doing this has profoundly affected my whole life, and I am eternally grateful and want to spread the word so that others may experience its magic. I was so blown away by my experience and what I saw in others that when I lived in New Zealand, I supported courses in my town. It was a wonderful, magical, fulfilling experience. For me, the path of Ascension has truly been a path of joy, love, compassion, gratitude, and so much more. No longer do the gremlins in my head plague me. No more do I want to get out of here. No more do I attach and hold on for dear life to the thoughts that led me to despair, loneliness, isolation, fear, and anger. No longer do I ruminate for hours or have sleepless nights with worry. I no longer feel the pressure of being too busy to the point of having palpitations as I once did. I do not compare myself to others or wish I had what someone else has. I don't dwell on past hurtful events that once ruled my days and led me to choices that hurt me even more. I no longer question what life is about or if there is more to life. I am not looking to be happy when... Which I used to say quite frequently when my kids were younger. I am no longer addicted to being right, proving someone else wrong!

The freedom that comes with no longer thinking I had to be a certain way is genuinely life-enhancing and life-changing. Life is filled with a richness I could never have imagined in my younger years. The whole dynamic of my family and friendships has been enhanced tenfold.

The beautiful, exciting, fun, joyous road to Ascension gave me the peace I had never experienced in my whole life. It brought me to my true self. I was allowing myself the freedom to be my unique self. I absolutely love that.

Where is your peace???

PART SIX
ASCENSION MEDITATION

'A Mindful Choice' is a film worth your time to watch. You can find it on 'The Bright Path' website, where you can watch it for free.

Ascension meditation is taught by Ishaya's of The Bright Path. It is a traditional teaching which goes back many centuries. Ishaya are modern-day monks who dedicate their lives to maintaining the traditional teachings of those who have gone before them. The initial training is called The First Sphere and is conducted over a weekend.

It is a transformational weekend.

You can find first sphere teachings also on 'The Bright Path' website and many wonderful articles written by the Ishaya's.

Looking back on my life now after learning and living Ascension, I acknowledge that too much of my life was lived in unnecessary underlying fear and anxiety. Mum having a nervous breakdown, Dad leaving so abruptly at a time when our home was also taken, then re-marrying and creating another life for himself, leaving us behind, and so many more stories from childhood shaped some very disruptive behaviour in my sisters and me. All of the hurt appeared the more vulnerable I became through menopause. Taking on responsibilities way above my age or ability. I aged quickly, took things far too seriously, built friendships around how I could solve others' problems, and could not acknowledge any of my own needs. I wanted so much to know that I was loved and to have the freedom of a fun childhood. The burden of life weighed me down, and I certainly felt it. I took charge efficiently and effectively and became the one everyone else turned to. I was a real hero, and my self-worth became based on it. I found it incredible that all this hurt was right there with me in menopause.

When I discovered Ascension through the film 'A Mindful Choice' produced by Greg Hopkins and Sally Lewis (their Ishaya names are Mahakala and Aditi. You will see Aditi's story through menopause later in

PART SIX
ASCENSION MEDITATION

this chapter), so many of the burdens fell away quickly. My attitude to life changed profoundly and beautifully.

To allow peace instantly into your life, let go of the:

Gossip

Family arguments

The need to be the centre of attention.

The need to conform to the expectations of others.

The need to prove you're right.

The need to please everyone.

The need to prove yourself.

Fully embrace:

Your values

MENOPAUSE MIND SHIFTS

Your vision

Your dreams

Your life

Your peace

Ascension meditation was the first tool in my toolbox that quickly led me to experience peace and stillness within myself for the first time in my life. I can pinpoint the exact moment that I felt entirely peaceful. Completely still. Like a feather gently floating on the breeze, Ascension gave me what I needed at the time I needed it the most. It turned my menopause journey on its head. It gave me a complete sense of joy and a new love for everything I was experiencing. I couldn't believe how light I felt. It was as if I were wearing a new pair of glasses and could see my world from many angles with much more clarity. All I had to do once I had learned the techniques was to keep doing it and commit 100%. Not 98 or 99 %. Committed 100%, no questions

PART SIX
ASCENSION MEDITATION

asked, no doubts or fears. I felt peace, and I wanted more of it. I was determined to "prioritise my peace" firstly for my sake, but I quickly saw how it rippled out to my family, friends, clients, and staff. "Prioritise my peace" became my new mantra to live by, and I loved it. Ascension meditation taught by Ishaya's of The Bright Path could be your pivotal point in finding wellness within the horrors of menopause. The experience changed my inner world. It dramatically calmed my nervous system.

Some beautifully written words from women who Ascend.

JAYA:

The practice of ascension clearly has shown me that I can watch whatever is happening in my mind, body, and world.

By watching it, I have the freedom to experience it, but not to then worry about it.

MENOPAUSE MIND SHIFTS

What happens in "my" mind is probably similar to what can happen in your mind.

I can think up and judge and assume an entirely new world. It can be a dark world filled with worry and fear or a daydream world of the perfect fantasy.

But when it came to my health, I could think as if I were a doctor convincing myself of my pending illness.

A change in my monthly period and then the change with the hot flushes as menopause crept in, and I was already deadly ill and with little time left.

That's what my mind was saying!

I feel blessed that with the practice of The Bright Path, I have developed a firm knowingness and natural identification with resting in this present moment.

This ability to be in the present moment has allowed me to see the thoughts as unreal and definitely not me.

PART SIX
ASCENSION MEDITATION

I can watch with fascination the changes in my body. I love the body and know it has an intelligence that "I" don't understand.

This beautiful dance of seeing what's passing... and sometimes getting caught in it by thinking about it is something which amazes me.

Nothing is right or wrong, but the dance of watching and seeing.

The body isn't right or wrong for hot flushes, sudden emotions, or menopausal changes... but with my ability to be present, I don't see it as an intense or challenging stage of my life.

I would like my husband to write and share because he might see my changes differently.

What I don't know and appreciate so much is that my husband and I have created a very conscious relationship where we don't judge and attack each other.

I can't imagine that.

So, if I was experiencing weird menopausal changes, my husband had the ability not to take things personally but to share honestly if he didn't think that way of acting was appropriate.

So, I look to him for that clarity if I'm having a moment of in-clarity... and I feel it is a blessing to have that.

My Dance with Menopause

By: Aditi - Ishaya Monk & Teacher of Ascension Meditation

In my early 40's, I was fresh out of a marriage and on the path to rediscovering myself. Well... that's what I told myself anyway, but secretly, I didn't know what that really meant. Seventeen years with Paul, my husband, hadn't been a disaster by any means. We'd actually been good together and happy for much of that time; but not towards the end. We both knew we weren't making each other happy and that it was time to 'gift' each other our freedom. I'd somehow lost my self-confidence and

PART SIX
ASCENSION MEDITATION

identity, and I could see it in Paul's eyes when he looked at me. I think he wanted to help me get back to my old, vibrant self as much as I did, but we knew we couldn't do it together.

It was scary at times to imagine what my future might look like, but mostly, I had a feeling of excitement with the new possibilities that might come my way. New adventures to be had, and one of those new adventures I quickly discovered was menopause!

Paul and I hadn't had children, so I had this preconceived idea that I would skip lightly through menopause, entering my 50s as a confident, free-spirited woman, fully equipped for the next chapter of my life. My mother and older sister had never shared anything about their experience, so I thought it must have been a breeze for them, too. I observed 50-something women; they seemed to have a vibrancy about them that I didn't yet possess, so I assumed that aliveness would be the glorious byproduct of any physical discomfort I might have to go through.

How wrong was I!

It came as a shock when I started having fortnightly periods in my early forties and hot flushes every 20 minutes, day and night! Blankets on, blankets off, blankets on… I was forever premenstrual or post-menstrual, with a couple of days in between where I felt slightly 'normal', although I was very quickly losing sight of what 'normal' was. Lack of sleep on its own definitely made me into something less than pretty.

My doctor, who could have brushed up on his bedside manner, informed me that my blood tests showed I was only 'perimenopausal' (you've got to be joking!) and that there was nothing he could do. "You just have to learn to live with it" were his parting words, which was rather devastating for a 'more than slightly' depressed woman lacking any kind of normal sleep pattern. I didn't cry a lot or have

PART SIX
ASCENSION MEDITATION

massive mood swings, but I did hide my depression as if it were a curse. A friend recommended I try a Family Planning doctor who was a lot more helpful and understanding. An option was going on HRT (Hormone Replacement Therapy), but I wanted to avoid that if I could, so I tried more natural remedies. They helped a little, but I finally succumbed and used HRT for three months solely to catch up on sleep. It worked. Some semblances of normality returned, but the hot flushes continued.

My Thought Patterns

Through all of this, there was something happening within me that was more disturbing. Nothing prepared me for the internal dialogue, the intense thoughts and the mind chatter that came along with the changes I was experiencing physically. Nobody ever mentioned that wee gem of a side effect. And at the time, I made no correlation between menopause and my increasingly gnarly inner voices. It wasn't until Deb shared her story with me over coffee one day, only recently, that I understood why my mind had switched gears so violently through my 40s. Thank you, Deb, for writing this book and helping raise awareness. I'm sure if I'd read this book in my forties, I would have had a lot more understanding and gentleness towards myself and what I was about to go through.

Our loved ones and the people around us are very aware of the outward symptoms of menopause; the hot flushes, the mood swings, the irritability - but the inner, self-violent thinking seemed to creep up on me and take over every aspect of my life before I even noticed it. It certainly wasn't something I wanted to admit to anyone.

It was such a gradual shift that I had just assumed it was 'me' getting older. Even though I thought I had a very convincing outward persona of a happy, well-balanced, successful businesswoman (which was getting much harder to maintain by this stage), my internal chatter had led me to a total lack of inner self-confidence; anxiety; depression; an

PART SIX
ASCENSION MEDITATION

inability to make decisions; a mistrust of everything around me including myself, and an ever-increasing feeling of discontent. Literally, fear had displaced the boldness of my youth!

The thoughts were sometimes subtle; other times, they were so in my face that it felt like another woman was living inside of me, and she'd taken over my life. She just wouldn't shut up. And she was sooo mean! She judged me constantly; she judged others as less than me, and there was always something wrong. Something wrong with 'me', something wrong with my outside world. Of course, those downward spiralling patterns of thinking created very unsatisfactory patterns of behaviour that greatly impacted my experience of life. But the most frightening and destructive pattern was my constant self-criticism. Life just wasn't fun anymore.

I had no clue who I was, and it was time to take action. I read heaps of books about consciousness and the power of being present. I did self-help and empowerment courses trying to reveal peace and be happy and had a series of visits with an empathetic and capable psychologist. They all helped me understand myself more and how my past had impacted my present, but I always got to a point where I slipped back into the old patterns. I thought I was still 'broken' somehow and just hadn't found the magic pill that would make it all right again. There had to be more to life than what I was experiencing. As I look back, I was facing my own mortality, perhaps for the very first time—and I needed help.

Questions like 'Who Am I?', 'Why Am I Here?', and 'What's the meaning of life?' kept floating around in my head. I'd heard those questions so many times that they sounded unanswerable and glib, but I was determined to persevere. Everything I'd done so far gave me plenty of insights into the idea of 'freedom from the mind', this present moment, a spiritual path, but nothing gave me an actual, direct experience of it. Staring at a leaf or watching a gorgeous sunset was about the extent of

PART SIX
ASCENSION MEDITATION

my ability to be present. Fleeting at best and definitely not sustainable. It's hard to carry a leaf around with you all day, so you can stare longingly at it whenever you want some peace. Besides, someone might put me away for that kind of behaviour!

I knew there was something more—the missing piece/peace, the meaning of life, freedom from my mind. I just knew it. I had to find a way to experience it and knew it had something to do with being present and here now.

Coming To Ascension Meditation

When it was suggested I learn to meditate using the Ishayas' Ascension techniques, I approached it in part to try and mitigate the physical symptoms of menopause, as I'd heard it might help. But more importantly, I needed to quieten the inner voices. To 'know me' again. Not the gnarly woman who was always irritable and looking for the next thing to go wrong but that vibrant woman I'd been in my early

20s, traveling the world without a care. The real 'me'.

I was very sceptical that it would actually work. My mind said it wasn't for me, but to be honest, I'd tried everything else, so why not give this a go? Tiredness and depression, hot flushes every 20 minutes, day and night, were all something I desperately wanted to change my relationship with. Ascension offered the hope of some small respite.

I had the idea that meditation was some weird spiritual practice that would take me to some different place. I thought of angels and out-of-body experiences—which didn't make much sense or hold much interest for me. I also had a fear of religion and brainwashing! Luckily, Ascension meditation was none of those things and was so much more practical and effective that I could be calm and choose for that any time I wanted. I felt like a child again, free from the limitations of the voices in my head.

PART SIX
ASCENSION MEDITATION

'Yes, it made me feel more connected to a greater force for good or a higher power. Still, more importantly, it gave me a mechanical way to disengage my mind and the voices in my head that were constantly pulling me into the past or projecting worry and anxiety into the future. In its simplicity, it revealed the present moment. A still, silent space, just beyond the movement of the mind, that was a natural state of peace and an overwhelming sense of well-being. Along with it naturally came more joy, more contentment. My mind was finally my life.

It didn't mean that I had no thoughts. It just meant that I could let them come and let them go. They didn't have the hold over me they had had in the past. I could feel the emotion of frustration with my tenth hot flush for the morning, but I could watch it and see it disappear. Finally, I had changed my relationship with thoughts, and my mind was calm.

Allowing

MENOPAUSE MIND SHIFTS

One of my greatest discoveries from meditating regularly was to find that 'Resistance Is Futile'! 'Allowing' is everything. Allowing the inner experience to be as it is, allowing emotions and internal chatter to move through rather than resisting or trying to control them. From there, more peace, joy and contentment sprung forth; no matter what was happening with my body.

My body was going to do what it was going to do. I could either resist it every step of the way or go along for the ride. Accepting or allowing my situation to be as it was, wasn't a passive thing either. It was a moment-by-moment choice to be present in life and to embrace all experiences.

In essence, I was changing my relationship to my thoughts, and I had the tools to move my attention elsewhere, away from the appearance of pain and suffering. And I liked it!

That didn't mean I didn't visit my doctor or go on HRT for three months so I could get some sleep, but

PART SIX
ASCENSION MEDITATION

I wasn't fighting it anymore. I was at peace with my body changes and my mental gymnastics. From there, actions or intuitive solutions appeared. The hot flushes didn't change in frequency for a while, but my relationship with them did—their intensity diminished when I was present with them. They didn't need to stop or even slow down for me to be at peace. That brought a different kind of focus to my life and an immense amount of peace and contentment. I started to feel human again.

Ascension helped me discover who I really am and who I want to be. It enabled me to live my purpose and open my mind to new experiences with less resistance and greater ease. Letting go of control, being gentle with myself, and allowing my experience to be as it was were major contributors to my experience of happiness.

It enabled me to perceive everything, including my thoughts, from a totally different perspective.

Letting Go Of Control

Another significant discovery was that 'I am not in control'—of anything. That was a huge discovery for an A+ control freak like me and, weirdly, very freeing. I'd spent my entire adult life trying to control everything—myself, my partner, the people and situations in my life, the outcomes. I was exhausted. It was a huge relief that I didn't need to control my menopause, let alone anything else. I didn't believe it at first, but with the consistent use of the Ascension techniques, letting go became a stable experience.

Other Women I've Taught To Meditate

Before I learned to Ascend, I had the belief that my thoughts were so terrible that I couldn't share them and that they were far worse than anyone else's thoughts. People would be horrified or reject me if they knew what was happening inside my head. How wrong was I! I've been teaching meditation for the past ten years and have seen so many women come along with the same mental

PART SIX
ASCENSION MEDITATION

'symptoms' that I experienced through menopause. We are so similar in our limiting, downward-spiralling beliefs about ourselves, yet we are so often too afraid to share them with anyone. Regular meditation made me realise I was far more connected to life than I'd ever imagined. This helped dissolve the sense of a separate 'me', and it helped me experience more connectedness with others.

I'd always thought my mental distress was a by-product of getting older and that I was alone. I also thought that women naturally worried more, got more anxious, put themselves in a smaller and smaller box, and felt more fearful of life as they aged.

Did I put that down to menopause? No, I didn't—not until Deb and I had our conversation over coffee that day. Knowing it's probably due to menopause is at least comforting and knowing that the voices in our heads aren't permanent is truly liberating.

MENOPAUSE MIND SHIFTS

Do I understand why we must go through this discomfort? No, I don't. Do I need to understand? No, I don't. It doesn't matter to me anymore. I'm just so thankful I found effective tools to be at peace with whatever is happening without judgment. To be able to handle whatever life dishes up with grace and dignity. Becoming aware of our thought patterns is the first step to letting them go. Finding an effective tool to let them go is the next step.

My 50s did indeed end up vibrant, exciting and magical—and definitely not what I expected! I got so hooked on meditation and my experience of life that I became an Ishaya monk one month after my 50th birthday. 'Ishaya' is a Sanskrit word that means 'For Higher Consciousness'. The Ishaya monks of The Bright Path are devoted to helping others experience more peace and a higher state of human consciousness. I have committed my life to helping raise the level of consciousness on the planet, to help people recognise that suffering is not obligatory! We all have a choice between peace and

PART SIX
ASCENSION MEDITATION

pain. Having the right tools and the right approach is essential.

I've recently hit 60, and I'm moving into a new decade with awe and excitement—living life fully, one moment at a time.

I wish you all the best on your journey through life and encourage you to find an effective meditation tool that suits you, to help you move along the road to freedom and a life fully lived.

More Resources

If you are interested in Ascension as taught by the Ishayas' of The Bright Path, you can find more at www.thebrightpath.com

Ascension is a non-religious, mechanical tool that can be used with eyes open, and eyes closed.

A survey of 2000 people revealed that:

MENOPAUSE MIND SHIFTS

97% of people who regularly use the Ascension meditation techniques report more peace, love and joy in their lives.

PART SEVEN
A WOMEN'S ADVICE

Author Unknown.

I asked a friend who has crossed 70 & is heading towards 80 what changes she feels in herself. She sent me the following:

1. After loving my parents, my siblings, my spouse, my children, and my friends, I have now started loving myself.
2. I have realised that I am not an "Atlas" ...

The world does not rest on my shoulders.

PART SEVEN
A WOMEN'S ADVICE

3. I have stopped bargaining with vegetable & fruit vendors. A few pennies more is not going to break me, but it might help the poor fellow save for his daughter's school fees.

4. I leave my waitress a big tip. The extra money might bring a smile to her face. She is toiling much harder for a living than I am.

5. I stopped telling the elderly that they've already narrated that story many times. The story makes them walk down memory lane & relive their past.

6. I have learned not to correct people even when I know they are wrong. The onus of making everyone perfect is not on me. Peace is more precious than perfection.

7. I give compliments freely & generously. Compliments are a mood enhancer not only for the recipient but also for me. And a small tip for the recipient of a compliment, never, NEVER turn it down; just say "Thank You."

MENOPAUSE MIND SHIFTS

8. I have learned not to bother about a crease or a spot on my shirt. Personality speaks louder than appearances.
9. I walk away from people who don't value me. They might not know my worth, but I do.
10. I remain cool when someone plays dirty to outrun me in the rat race. I am not a rat & neither am I in any race.
11. I am learning not to be embarrassed by my emotions. It's my emotions that make me human.
12. I have learned that it's better to drop the ego than to break a relationship. My ego will keep me aloof, whereas, with relationships, I will never be alone.
13. I have learned to live each day as if it's the last. After all, it might be the last.
14. I am doing what makes me happy. I am responsible for my happiness, and I owe it to myself. Happiness is a choice. You can be happy at any time; just choose to be!

PART SEVEN
A WOMEN'S ADVICE

I decided to share this with all my friends. Why do we have to wait to be 60 or 70, or 80? Why can't we practice this at any stage and age?

What advice would you give your daughters, ladies?

Conclusion

I truly believe that Women need Women. It is so important to have other beautiful women in your life. Who could possibly understand you the way other women could understand you?

'I sat quietly in the chair by the side of the hospital bed, watching my beautiful baby girl sleeping peacefully. The trauma of her birth not fazing her at all.

Every part of my body is swollen, and I'm exhausted. The blood transfusion needle still in my arm provides yet another unit of blood that drips

CONCLUSION

slowly and steadily. I sit, hoping this will give me some energy to be able to hold her close.

It's almost visiting time. I don't want to be seen like this. I have no energy for niceties. No willpower to push through. How can having a baby, one of the most exciting times in a woman's life, be so catastrophically traumatic? I can hardly keep my eyes open from the swelling or move my body from the exhaustion, so I sleep.

When I open my eyes, my friend is looking at me from the doorway. Our eyes meet. Nothing is said as we both begin to cry softly. Nothing needs to be said. In that very precious moment, she sees me in all my vulnerability, and I know she understands.

Women need women.

To this day, I will always remember that sense of pure relief for being seen and understood in all my complete vulnerability. Nothing needed to be said. When I see other women of a similar age, I see signs of menopause. I see them. I understand their struggles with life, maintaining their dignity, their relationships, their careers, and their appearance, and my heart bursts with wanting to help in any way I can.

Women need women. We are beautiful, intuitive beings who are truly magnificent when we allow ourselves to be who we are. In today's world, many women are lost. Lost in analytical thinking, being task-focused, rushing from one thing to the next to prove themselves. We have lost our ability to tune into our intuition, use our creativity, listen to our bodies, and approach things softly and gently, allowing our emotions to flow.

At the point at which menopause enters our lives, we would do well to tune back into those things that make a woman so special and let go of trying to fit into a male-dominated world. To see each other and hold each other in all our vulnerability, knowing that

CONCLUSION

inside, we have our own personal power beyond anything we could imagine.

My deepest desire is that by the time you have reached the end of this book, you are now better equipped to understand your own needs. That you have new knowledge about yourself that will better your life moving forward. That you have re-written some old limiting beliefs into vibrant, new, exciting ones that lift your life to newer heights. Maybe you have shed a tear as I have when writing as I realised something new that allowed me to release the pain I have unknowingly held for years. Profound realisations that hadn't occurred to me before and that shifted my perspective to something so much more positive and compassionate towards myself and others.

Maybe you have realised that it is OK to put yourself first and that in doing so, you are not being selfish. You matter; your life matters as much as all the people around you. You have every right to voice your opinions, speak your truth, rest when you need to, and let go of things that you no longer hold dear. You have every right to rid yourself of the labels you unknowingly accepted from others.

I hope you have realised that to blame only keeps you stuck in repeated patterns of behaviour that don't serve you. That whatever situation has caused you harm only comes from someone else's pain, and we only have a certain skill set to deal with what we experience in any given moment. Forgiveness and compassion are key for yourself and others.

As you place this book back on the shelf, can you give yourself lifetime permission to prioritise your peace, slow the pace of your life to give yourself space to tune into what is your own truth, the truth of who you are and what you truly want out of your life? To speak your truth always and allow your intuition to reveal itself. To slow life down enough to love and respect yourself and appreciate the contribution you make. Would this not be the best

CONCLUSION

gift you could teach your daughters as well as give to yourself?

To know that you are enough. Always have been and always will be.

The Japanese call menopause 'the second spring.' How beautiful! I certainly never thought of it as that when I was feeling at my worst. The second spring of new beginnings, new growth, new adventures. Who are you going to be? Who are you going to become? How has the information in this book changed your thoughts, your values, and your beliefs?

Embrace the life you are given and choose to live full out.

I love this quote:

> *"Life should not be a journey*
> *to the grave with the intention of*
> *arriving safely in a pretty and*
> *well-preserved body, but rather*

MENOPAUSE MIND SHIFTS

to skid in broadside in a cloud of smoke, thoroughly used up, totally worn out, and loudly proclaiming "Wow! What a Ride!!"

Hunter S. Thompson

I give you full permission to free yourself of limitation, of perceived perfectionism, and no longer allow yourself to just fit in and conform. Allow yourself the freedom of expression in whatever form feeds your soul and do this from a place of stillness and peace within your body. Stop. Look around. Allow stop-and-stare moments when you see a beautiful scene. Soak it up and repeatedly feed your heart and soul. Know who you are. Know what you want and go and get it. Fill your life to overflowing with love and compassion, joy, peace, and gratitude. You are worthy of every moment.

I truly hope you enjoyed reading this book as much as I have loved writing it. It has taken me on

CONCLUSION

a journey through my life memories and discoveries I would never have made had I not chosen to sit down and write. It has enabled me to heal relationships and re-frame experiences that have kept me trapped for most of my life.

Menopause robs so many women of a vibrant, healthy life. Let's keep spreading the word, have those conversations, and make the topic of menopause high on the agenda for the health and wellness of women around the world and for generations to come.

Thank you, beautiful soul, for buying this book.

Sending you all my love on your journey ahead

Deb

xxx

Resources

Fabulous books I would recommend to you.

'Menopausing' by Davina McCall with Dr Naomi Potter

'Women Thrive' by Raimonda Jankunaite, with contributions from other women who have faced adversity.

'Jump and your life will appear' by Nancy Levin

'200% An instruction manual for living fully' by Arjuna Ishaya

RESOURCES

'Cracking the Menopause - While keeping yourself together' by Mariella Frostrup & Alice Smellie

'The Menopause Reset' by Dr Mindy Pelz

'Breaking the Habit of Being Yourself' by Dr. Joe Dispenza

'Change your thoughts Change your Life' by Dr Wayne Dyer

'Big Magic' by Elizabeth Gilbert

'New Beginnings' by Sandy C. Newbigging

Acknowledgements

To my wonderful sister Becky for always encouraging me to strive for the best version of myself, for believing in me and inspiring me, and for always being there when I need someone to lean on. I love you, Sis, and I'm so grateful to have you so close in my life. Thank you for your photo cover for the book. What a creative talent you are.

To my beautiful sister Dulcie. This book has taken me on a journey I was unaware of. I love you and admire you from afar in the hope that one day, we can reconnect and let go of the pain and expectations caused by our childhood. I love you for

ACKNOWLEDGEMENTS

being the rock that you are and the security you have always provided for Mum.

Mum and Dad, my life would not exist without you both. For all the trials and tribulations that have made me who I am today, I am grateful. I can look back and see all the good that you instilled in us. How you showed us to value the simple things in life. I love you both for all that you are and all that you have taught me.

Kath and Hans, you are the best mother and father-in-law I could ever have wished for. Thank you so much for supporting me with my education in those early years and for being the best role models Dave and I could have in how to love each other unconditionally, grasp life with both hands and live fully. I love you both so much and will always be grateful for your guidance.

Aunty Sue at a time in my life when I needed support, comfort, a safe place to come to it was you who provided that for me. I love your fun filled, get out there and do it approach to life. I'm so lucky to have you in my life. Thank you for all that you have done for me. Thankyou for being a strong female role model in my life. I love you x

Aditi and Mahakala, my life changed for the better when I met you and the Ishaya's of The Bright Path. I am forever grateful for your teachings of the stillness I now experience in my life through Ascension meditation practice.

So many amazing people have influenced me on my journey to this point in my life.

Thank you to Sharon Pearson and The Coaching Institute, Melbourne; I have learnt so much from your amazing teachings.

Carrie Green from Female Entrepreneur Association UK. Your passion for helping other women succeed is infectious. I love sitting down for a Carrie uplifting, down-to-earth clarity session.

ACKNOWLEDGEMENTS

Lisa Johnson Business Strategist UK. I have learnt so much from you, Lisa, and I love your story, from childhood adversity to success. You have been such an inspiration from afar. I love how you can have such an impact on my life, and yet you have no idea who I am.

Nigel Botterill and the team from Entrepreneur Circle UK, I love being a member. Thank you for all your guidance and dedication to our entrepreneurial success.

To Reid Tracey (CEO of Hay House Publishers) and Kellie Notaras (KN Literary agents) for creating Authorprenuer Membership and helping me to believe I could bring this book to life.

Raimonda Jankunaite, founder of Women Thrive and all the women who are willing and able to share their life stories of vulnerability and success. I am so grateful for the opportunity to speak on your stage.

For all our friends in New Zealand and the incredible experiences we have had living in another country.

My life would not be complete without the love of my life and our wonderful young humans and, of course, Woody, our dog. Pendle and Roo, even though you are not with us, you are always in our hearts. I love you all so completely.

About The Author

Dear reader

I thought I would share a little more about myself. I am from Lancashire in the UK. In 2006, my husband and I decided we wanted an adventure. So, we sold our home, packed our belongings and two very young children, and headed for the beautiful country of New Zealand. What a wonderful life-enriching experience it was to live in another country, another culture. We learned so much about ourselves during this time.

In 2022, it was time to come home. To return to our own people and our culture with a totally new perspective on our homeland. I have the deepest love and admiration for both countries, the friends we have, and the experiences we encountered.

I absolutely love being in nature, walking in the rain, writing, coaching people to discover the life they want to live, cosying up to my hubby to watch a great English drama, having good nourishing food shared with family and friends, and watching the kids cook. The simplest things in life fill me with pure joy.

I learned to create the life I love living every single day. I love my husband, my kids, my friends, our dog Woody and our cats Pendle and Roo. I love my sisters, my parents, and my parents-in-law. A life filled with love is a life well lived.

I figured out how to be 'supremely gentle' and that, filling my life with love, stillness, joy, and, as Arjuna Ishaya puts it, living life 100% on the outside, 100% on the inside, I created the life I wanted to live. I discovered I had choices. So, I choose to live fully, and I choose that NOW. Being with this wonderful thing called life, moment by moment, is a very special and precious way to live. Anyone can do it.

The journey of writing this book has been one filled with emotion and love. A deeper journey of self-discovery and a release of hurt I knew one day would need to come out. The journey is worth it for the freedom within that it gives you.

So, with my memories and thoughts out into the world, I will carry on my journey with an open heart filled with curiosity and love for my life as it unfolds. I hope you can do the same and that this book has given you the awareness you need.

From my heart and soul to yours, with love

Deb

About Soul Decisions Coaching

Soul Decisions Coaching is a joint venture between sisters Debbie and Becky.

Deb is a qualified Occupational Therapist (OT) with 30-plus years of experience in the health service both in the UK and New Zealand. Her experience took her from working in Paediatrics to Adult Palliative and End of Life Care. Deb is now a registered OT in the UK, working predominantly as a Life Coach and Bowen Therapist with women of menopausal age who want to re-energize

ABOUT SOUL DECISIONS COACHING

themselves and their relationships and reclaim their lives.

Becky Kelly is a passionate advocate for natural health and wellness. She is a certified practitioner of Bowen Therapy, a gentle and effective technique that stimulates the body's innate healing response. She is also a Dr. Sears certified Health and Wellness Coach with over ten years of experience in guiding clients to make positive lifestyle changes. Becky has a particular interest in gut health, as she understands the vital role that the digestive system plays in overall well-being. She offers comprehensive gut health support using Bowen Therapy and Coaching. She also provides personalised nutrition and supplement recommendations to support optimal gut function and microbiome balance. Becky believes that everyone deserves to live a pain-free and fulfilling life, and she is committed to providing personalised and compassionate coaching and therapy services at Soul Decisions Coaching.

MENOPAUSE MIND SHIFTS

To find out more about us and what we have to offer, please visit our website:

www.souldecisionscoaching.com

Or email:

deb@souldecisionscoaching.com

rebecca@souldecisionscoaching.com

We would love to hear from you!

XX

Other Titles by Soul Decisions Coaching

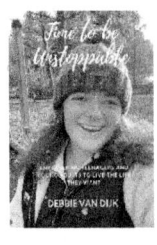

Time to Be Unstoppable. Empowering Teenagers and Young Adults To Live The Life They Want. By Deb van Dijk

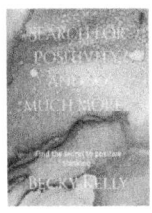

Search for Positivity and so much more...: Find the secret to positive thinking. By Becky Kelly

MENOPAUSE MIND SHIFTS

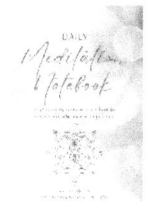
Daily Meditation Notebook. A 90-day daily meditation notebook to capture your subconscious inspirations. By Becky Kelly

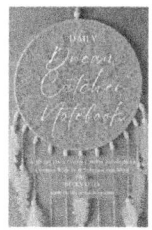
Daily Dream Catcher Notebook. A 30-day daily dream catcher notebook to Connect With Your Subconscious Mind. By Becky Kelly

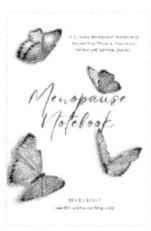
Menopause Notebook. A 12-week Menopause Notebook to Record Your Physical, Emotional, Mental, and Spiritual Journey. By Becky Kelly

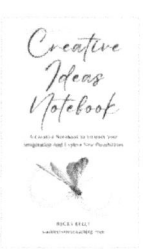
Creative Ideas Notebook. A Creative Notebook to Unleash Your Imagination And Explore New Possibilities. By Becky Kelly

OTHER TITLES BY SOUL DECISIONS COACHING

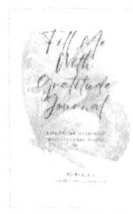

Fill Me With Gratitude Journal. A place for you to express the things you are truly thankful for. By Becky Kelly

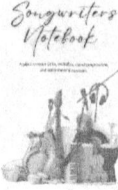

Songwriters Notebook. A place to store lyrics, melodies, chord progressions, and other musical concepts. By Becky Kelly

See our books on our website:

www.souldecisionscoaching.com

Printed in Great Britain
by Amazon